Jailhouse Shrink

A How-To Manual

On Practicing Psychiatry in Jails

Fourth Edition

Edward Hume MD

Table of Contents

Forward:
Jailhouse Shrink –
A How-to Manual

Background

This is a nonacademic how-to manual on practicing psychiatry in jails. You already know how to do psychiatry. This is about doing it in jails.

Why practice psychiatry in jails? Aren't jails dangerous places? Aren't jails part of the immoral apparatus our society uses to oppress the poor? Why contribute to the oppression?

Actually, properly done, jails are the safest place to practice. Going from other practice settings to inpatient care you might be shocked at how dangerous psychiatric hospitals have become. You will be ever so happy to get to the safety of jails.

Our jails are crowded. They are full of people waiting for court. They are also full of mentally ill people. If you are committed to treating psychiatrically disturbed individuals, where can you make more of a difference than in a jail?

Most of the "victims" you see are victimizers. Some are innocent of wrongdoing. Our courts are slow. People are arrested, guilt undetermined, only to languish long, waiting for their day in court. Yet the lawyers—first one side, then the other—ask for delay after delay; and those delays are granted. If you are too poor to make bail, you can literally wait years in jail waiting for some court to recognize that they arrested the wrong guy, for example. So isn't taking care of people in jail a way of participating in an unjust system? (Yes, it is true in some states that by abolishing bail, people in theory are not held because they have no money. But there are still injustices.)

However unjust the system may be, some inmates still need care. They are under enormous stress, confined in a mix of criminals, drug addicts, and normal people. The circumstances of confinement are hard, sometimes cruel. After all, confinement is a form of punishment.

Pretrial detention can be seen as a form of pre-guilt punishment. Courts tacitly acknowledge this when they release guilty persons with a sentence of "time served." People confined in this way are unhappy and can become depressed; they may need treatment. Others are unable to cope with confinement; they need to be diagnosed and appropriately treated. Here is where the medical practitioner skilled in psychiatric diagnosis and treatment is badly needed, no matter if the system is just or unjust.

Practicing psychiatry in jails is different from practicing psychiatry "on the street;" that is, in your private practices. You basically have to throw out a lot of what you do and start all over again from the first principals of practicing medicine. Especially, you can't just be a "happy pill" dispenser, distinguishable from the neighborhood drug dealer only by the kind of drugs you prescribe. In fact, in the case of benzodiazepines (e.g.—"Zannies," etc.), you give access to the same chemicals as the drug dealer; the only difference is that you require appointments and dispense prescriptions that must be filled at a drugstore. A drug dealer is far more convenient than you are.

One thing about working in jails: the tremendous variety of the cases you see. Your attention will be drawn to plain depression and psychotic disorders; drug addictions and covert brain injuries from TBI's. Keep an open mind and you will see a huge variety of clinical conditions. Not everyone has a "bipolar disorder."

Our job is to treat mental illness, not to give drugs to non-ill people simply because they are having a hard time coping with adverse circumstances. Doing that does them no favors. Thus psychiatric diagnosis in the jail setting involves distinguishing mental illness from mere distress and giving the inmate treatment appropriate for her illness while allowing the normal person the opportunity to cope.

Note that a jail is not a prison. Prison practice differs from jail practice, and requires a different approach. This book will cover jail practice. What follows is a brief overview on practicing psychiatry in jails, not prisons. It is not a cookbook, however. There is much discretion involved. You need to know your business as a prescriber. You have to know how to diagnose and treat mental and physical illness, before you can help anyone in a jail.

Circumstances

The jail is an interesting place. People who have committed crimes come to a jail; and people come to jail who have not committed crimes. They are locked down in anxiety-provoking situations. They are often too nervous to sleep very well; or they are appropriately vigilant and therefore sleep lightly. As such, you must weigh all of inmates' complaints in order to get a handle on whether you are dealing with an illness, or simply a normal reaction to tough circumstances.

A jail medical practice is also cost-constrained; we are required to practice cost-effective medicine (after all, taxpayers pay for everything we do). We don't do necessarily everything a person wants. Instead, we give them what they need. The best care may not mean the most recent "advances" in prescription drugs. In fact, the best care may be going back to what is old and cheap and works very well.

Even though a jail practice is cost-constrained if you work for a good company, you will not be afflicted by managed care or anything like it. Managed care companies make their profits from denying care. The managed care companies are supposed to allow appropriate care, but they harass psychiatrists who try to provide that appropriate care. Luckily, the companies that are contracted to provide care to inmates usually do not harass their providers. They simply want to get the job done with minimal hassle. You will probably find this to be quite refreshing.

Diagnosis

You must always start from scratch in making a diagnosis. Never accept someone else's diagnosis. We learned this long ago when we were changing psychiatry from a psychologically based field to a medically based one. The process of diagnosis has come a long way in that time. However, it has still yet a long way to go. So you must not trust your colleagues to provide you a diagnosis. Use somebody else's diagnosis as a starting point for asking questions. The one exception to this is when another practitioner has left enough detailed information that you can arrive at a diagnosis independently from the information your colleague provided. That colleague need not be a psychiatrist; he or she might be an APN, a psychologist or a counselor. You may supplement the workup with a few questions. In the event, you should make each diagnosis on your own so you can trust the diagnosis that you see in front of you. If this means rediagnosing each inmate, so be it.

Prescribing

In prescribing, always remember that you are in cost-constrained situation. Having costs constrained does not mean that you cannot prescribe the best medication. What cost-constrained care means is that you can't indulge yourself and prescribe whatever the most recent drug rep told you about. When you look at studies done on actual patients, these new miracle medications have a difficult time separating themselves from placebo. In many cases the best treatments are treatments that long ago became generic.

First-generation antipsychotics are becoming known as neurotoxic. Nonetheless, these are medications you must learn to use because in many cases these are the medications that work for a particular inmate.

Counseling

It may seem archaic and odd in this day of medical wonders, but counseling can do a far better job than many, many medications. Most of the inmates we see have difficulties with Attention Deficit Hyperactivity Disorder, Post-Traumatic Stress Disorder, Dysthymia, Borderline

Personality Disorder and Substance Abuse Disorders. They have many things which trouble them greatly. Frequently if they are taught the parameters of their difficulties, what to expect from their difficulties and how to overcome their difficulties, they can handle them on their own without necessarily needing someone to lead them by the hand.

The Model

Most of all you must understand the model of practicing psychiatry in a jail. Too often psychiatrists teach patients that every patient is helpless in the face of a biologically based illness; that the patient must take medications and come to see the psychiatrist on a regular basis or the patient will fall into sin and degradation; that they suffer from a "chemical imbalance;" that only the medication can rescue them from making terrible mistakes. Of course all of this is hogwash. The fact is what most often troubles inmates in jails is decisions they have made and the consequences of those decisions. By telling them that they are helpless, you give people of a criminal mindset an excuse not to take responsibility for their own behavior. If instead you will pay attention to the teachings of Alcoholics Anonymous, Narcotics Anonymous and the weightlifters, you will see these groups of people collectively know at least as much valuable clinical wisdom as all of psychiatry. Pay attention to what they have to teach us.

Education

Teachers in health classes seem to relish teaching young people how to put a condom on a banana. But they don't seem to teach the basic biology of the human body. Perhaps the most important thing you can teach an inmate is how the body releases and uses adrenaline, for example. See Appendix PA for specifics on panic attacks. But some inmates have health conditions they know little about. Other inmates are concerned about sleep but do not know anything about 'sleep hygiene.' They may think, for example, that waking at 9:50 in the morning after going to sleep at 2 AM is a problem. A little math tells you they are sleeping nearly 8 hours (real case). Basic instruction on taking care of their own bodies can go a long way in helping inmates.

The Chart and Clinical Notes

Your notes will go into what we physicians traditionally call a "chart." The chart is a collection of clinical records which include your notes. These days the "chart" may be a series of electronic notes which are grouped together because they have to do with a single inmate.

The purpose of clinical notes is communication across time. Although we traditionally understand it as communicating from one clinician to another, the note may be necessary to communicate to yourself a week, a month or a year after you have written it. It is important to make your note comprehensive enough that other people can understand what you meant and you can understand what you meant.

Even though we've been told over and over and over again that a chart is a legal document, the fact is it is only a legal document because the lawyers use the chart for legal purposes and because we need the notes in a chart to cover our rear ends when we're in legal trouble. The fact is that the chart is first and foremost a *clinical* document designed to communicate clinical information across time. The requirement of a "legal document" is that you keep in mind that a judge or a jury might be reading the material after you, so do a good job on your note.

Bottom Line

State governments have been shrinking their state hospitals while local governments have been expanding their jails. Cynics note that putting a person in a psychiatry unit or a mental hospital—perhaps because of its therapeutic focus—costs literally ten times as much as putting someone in a jail. Regardless of the reason, inmates in jail need to have psychiatric care available to them, and you will be there to provide it.

Remember that all around the country your profession is in short supply. More to the point, the jail has contracted for a minimal amount of your time. You must keep the load down so that you can see as many inmates as possible, and treat only those who really need treatment. You must not treat inmates' unhappiness; you treat their mental illnesses. Jail is a tough place for many people. **Inmates who have trouble coping need to learn how to cope.** You don't always help them by throwing pills at them.

And then there are the addicts. They arrange to see you because they want something to replace their drugs. It is not your job to cushion their detox. Anxiety and sleeplessness are symptoms of withdrawal and detoxification. Unless they have a preexisting psychiatric condition, addicts will do fine without medications from you.

Chapter 1
Welcome to Jail

Jails are the setting for a jailhouse psychiatric practice. If you work with inmates you will work at a jail, or in a prison or in a forensic hospital. All the settings differ from each other but the types of settings tend to clump together based on their missions. Forensic hospitals are there to treat people who are being assessed for competency or insanity, to figure out who is malingering, to treat the post-conviction mentally ill in particular and to treat the very dangerous mentally ill in general. Prisons are there to confine people convicted of felonies whether they have a mental illness or not. Jails, on the other hand, are a very mixed bag. They are designed to hold persons who have been arrested until they can stand trial or face a probationary hearing. They are also designed to hold people after they have been convicted of crimes. People who commit misdemeanors will typically "do" their time entirely in the jail. Felons are typically held until they can go off to prison. Some people are just waiting for their day in court when they will be sentenced to "time served" and released. And a few are innocent of any wrongdoing. Some or all these people have mental illness.

Jails have been around a long time. Over the decades and the centuries a technology has developed around the management of captive criminals, the overwhelming super–majority of people in jail. Over the years the management of inmates has evolved as the populations have changed and as the expectations of society have changed. Jails are not mired in the procedures of centuries past. Yet they remain true to their primary mission: they confine the people that society wants confined. When you think about it, psychiatric hospitals have a similar mission. So it should come as no surprise that as authorities have closed mental hospitals, more of their former inpatients become inmates in the correctional system.

Jails are designed to keep the public, civilian employees, the staff, and inmates safe, in that order. The architectural deficiencies of a jail are compensated by the procedures of correctional officers. They are the ones who make a facility safe for civilians like you, no matter how well or badly a jail is designed.

Jails are interesting places. More than prisons, they are human places. There is a society in each jail with an overall organization and a number of sub-societies (the medical department is one such sub-society). I'll leave it to you to discover the various sub-societies in your jail(s) but one group must be covered for it is crucial to the survival of everyone in jail: the Custody staff— the corrections officers, or CO's.

Corrections Officers

A corrections officer is not merely a guard. Calling a CO a "guard" is an insult. He is not there merely to guard the facility and the people in it. She is there to guard the facility and you, and to provide guidance to inmates so the inmates might move on to a less criminal life—hence the adjective "corrections." A CO has some authority and can issue instructions that inmates and we civilians must obey. So they are officers.

You will need to do more than get along with the CO's. You will need to work with Custody to get your job done. Always remember that you are working in their house. They set the rules. They establish the milieu. It is not your job to intercede on behalf of inmates against the custody staff. It is your job to help inmates cope with their circumstances. Inmates have grievance procedures far more powerful than anything you can accomplish. If you let yourself be persuaded to intervene on behalf of an inmate, you have been manipulated. You have been had.

Spend some time getting to know the CO's. Say hello when you see them. Learn their names. Look at them as your teammates. If you visit a pod to see inmates, ask the CO's what they have observed about inmate X, Y and Z. Consider it to be similar to asking nurses in a hospital what they have observed. You *do* ask nurses for their observations, right?

Most jails have ODRs—Officer Dining Rooms —where staff is served food. Try to have lunch in the ODR, always eat the jail staff food and sit with the CO's. Try not to sit with mental health or medical staff. You get to know each other, which is often a big help in doing your job. And sometimes a CO will tell you about an inmate who is flaking out, before he comes to your attention by normal channels. Better to catch something early, before it goes too far.

CO's are human. There are good CO's and bad CO's, lazy ones and diligent. But on the whole, CO's are hardworking and dedicated to their jobs. By providing an ever-present "cop on the beat" they keep the inmates in line and make jails safe to work in. But always be on the same team as the CO's. If you think of the CO's as your allies it is much easier to be civil, even friendly. A relaxed cheerful demeanor can do wonders in opening doors (sometimes literally) and getting things done. If CO's are glad to see you because you are glad to see them, things in general go ever so much better.

Security at the Front Gate

Most jails have open parking lots. Some jails have fenced lots with gates that are attended by guards (not CO's) or by CO's. Inside the front entrance of the building, but outside the secured spaces, there is always a security entrance where people who enter will be scanned for contraband before being allowed through to the jail proper. Some secured entrances are for all who enter— CO's, civilian staff, visitors. Some jails have different entrances for staff and visitors. Contraband always includes weapons—guns, knives, shivs, shanks. Sometimes it includes bags with opaque sides (you can actually buy purses with clear sides). Or maybe you cannot wear your coat inside. The one constant—aside from weapons—is the cell phone. You cannot bring one in. Cell phones are too useful to inmates for calling outside unsupervised. Inmates have been known to manage outside businesses or arrange for hits on the outside from the inside. So imagine my surprise when I was allowed at one of my jails to bring in a cell phone! What this proves is that every jail is different.

There is usually a logbook where you sign in. Or perhaps a logbook where the CO on duty notes that you are entering the building, and notes when you leave. The purpose of this logbook is twofold. First, it allows jail authorities to know who is entering and leaving their jail. More importantly, if some disaster strikes they know who is inside the building. So don't forget to sign in.

Most jails will issue you a security clearance. When you pass this, they will take your picture, obtain your fingerprints yet again and issue you an ID card. Or not. One jail I know used to have an ID card for me. Now they have a system where CO's look at you, familiarize themselves with you over several weeks, while you wear a temporary visitor's slip with your photograph. After a while, you are put on a list of approved civilians and allowed in. No more strangers with fake ID badges—the staff know you. But there are other jails that have simply procrastinated in issuing ID cards. You shrug your shoulders and work there anyway.

The advantage of an ID card, is that in some jails you have access to a locker inside the building but outside the security entrance. That way, you can wear a winter coat and cap inside the building and store it, entering staff spaces without such contraband and putting it away where someone will not walk off with it.

Interview Spaces

Each jail has its own setup for seeing inmates. The variety is astonishing. For example, you may interview inmates in an office that is "yours" for the day. You may walk around unit to unit to see inmates in a designated interview room on each unit. You may see inmates at a table in a common space where attorneys interview their clients. Although you may find yourself in a setting that is not directly supervised by a CO, most of the time CO's are watching while you interview the inmates. They may leave a door open so they can see you. They will follow their own procedures, but the main thrust is that it is their job to keep you safe.

The bottom line on jail procedures: there is more to them than we understand. The security staff has its priorities, and those center around 1) keeping society safe from inmates 2) keeping us non-custody staff—civilians—safe from inmates 3) keeping other inmates safe from inmates 4) keeping themselves safe from inmates and 5) all other issues (e.g.—Medical problems, mental health visits, attorney visits, etc.). It's Safety First, in layers.

So we can't expect anyone to cater to our needs as clinicians. We have to wait our turn. Consider that you must do what you advise inmates to do: wait, learn some patience, develop some humility.

Addendum: the Purpose of Jails

After this introduction you may be wondering why we have jails. After all, jails are a relatively recent phenomenon in our civilization. Before jails, we had lockups where people were held briefly before trial. People were punished with stocks, flogging and hanging. All were public. It is true there were a few people held in prisons, but these were generally held for reasons of state.

Jails are part of the legal process today. Jail has three functions: punishment, incapacitation and rehabilitation. Punishment is seen to serve three purposes, in no particular order: general deterrence, specific deterrence and retribution. General deterrence says to others "If you do that this will happen to you." Some research shows that punishment demonstrates to law-abiding citizens that they are not foolish to obey the laws. There are some people who will always follow the law. There are some people who will never follow the law. Most people are in the middle, more or less following the law, depending on the certainty and the severity of punishment. It is this vast middle who are responsive to general deterrence.

Specific deterrence says to the inmate "If you do that again, this punishment will happen to you again."

Retribution lets the general public know that the government is protecting their lives and property against malefactors. Retribution also serves to show the general public that adequate punishment was assessed, so that further punishment is not needed. Feuds are supposedly prevented this way (think of the Hatfields and the McCoys).

A lot of thought has gone into this and the thinking gets pretty deep, which is why the discussion was held to an addendum at the end of this chapter.

That detention in jail is supposed to serve the function of incapacitation, much as capital punishment used to do and occasionally still does.

That detention in jail is a form of punishment is clear when judges sentence people to time in jail as a consequence of committing a crime. For a poor person to languish in jail because he cannot make bail, when he may be innocent of any crime does not serve any of the purposes listed above (this explains "bail reform," or doing away with bail).

Further, when a severely mentally ill person is held in jail, few if any of society's goals are met. Take a schizophrenic. He doesn't care what day it is. He may remember that he has a hearing on a certain date but it doesn't register. Clearly, holding him in jail as a punishment for missing the hearing will not cause him to pay any better attention to the significance of dates. You can see the genesis of mental health courts here. (The problem with mental health courts is that once they exist, they become an escape hatch for criminals who are not mentally ill but know how to fake it. Wouldn't you like to be a judge?)

A person may be held for trial, as has always been the case. But when judges allow extensions of time in jail because an attorney is not ready or because a police officer can't make it, the process hardly seems fair to the defendant. If someone is a criminal, however, the "punishment" of jail time also serves to prevent his committing more crimes while he is detained. This is incapacitation. From that comes the complaint that police make against bail reform (i.e.—the elimination of bail): they get no break from criminal activity; criminals are not incapacitated.

The last function of a jail—and it is always last—is rehabilitation. While I have seen alcoholics dry out and drug addicts escape the influence of drugs while in jail, I have not seen a similar rehabilitation among straight criminals. Perhaps this is an artifact of perspective, and people do recover from a criminal lifestyle to become law-abiding citizens.

One can hope.

Chapter 2
The Clinical Population

Jails are where the police put people they don't want on your streets. These days when someone gets out of line they put him in jail first, ask questions later.

Of course the above is a bit of an exaggeration, but not by much. As a jailhouse shrink, you will be called upon to deal with whatever the cops dragged in. So let's see what we have.

First of all, you may have heard that jails are becoming substitutes for the psychiatric hospitals that governments are closing. While this is true, the population of mentally ill is not the largest group of inmates who want to see you and get chemicals from you. So, before you start prescribing medications to inmates, you need to understand your population. You will need to keep in mind the rule "First of all do no harm" in everything you do. It's a surprisingly easy rule to break, so you must work carefully.

Most people who come to jail have similar sets of characteristics, and generally share aspects of their personal history. You need to understand these groups of inmates and keep their characteristics in mind as you treat them.

ADHD and Substances

The largest group of people you will see had trouble sitting still and paying attention when young. They were easily distracted. They tended to resist going to bed at night, staying up late and perhaps needing little sleep. They did things suddenly without thinking first ('impulsive' is a fancy way of describing this). Often inmates, when asked about these characteristics, will say "Still do" or "That's why I'm here."

If you think I'm describing people labeled as ADHD you're right. But is it a disorder? Perhaps it is just a set of characteristics—like being tall—that exist more or less on a continuum. But however you conceive it, these characteristics can lead people to accomplish many things—negative and positive, if illegal.

The basis for long-term trouble our kids get into is substances—tobacco, marijuana, alcohol, cocaine, opiates and more. And this is big trouble. After you have worked in corrections a bit you will see many people who share the traumas of your office outpatients. So why are these inmates in jail and your office patients not? Usually the difference is drugs or alcohol.

Why is that? In short, you stop growing up when you start picking up. It is well known in NA and AA that people stop maturing when they start drinking or using drugs. And substance abuse counselors often remark after group sessions how immature—even boyish—the group members behave.

Let us imagine that growing up is like training to join a basketball team: you lift weights to get strong; you shoot baskets to practice your skills; you run laps to develop your endurance. But what happens if a machine lifts your weights for you? The weights get lifted but do you get strong? If your coach lets you use a basket-shooter during practice, the baskets get shot, but do you learn how to shoot baskets? And if I give you a motor scooter to ride around the track, you get around the track, but do you develop endurance?

I'm sure you can see where this is going. Adolescence is hard: you go from being a child to assuming the responsibilities of adulthood. Many unpleasant events occur, and the adolescent must learn to cope with them. Many tasks must be mastered. You come home after a hard day dealing with difficult people thinking to yourself "How could I have handled that better? How can I deal with an a_hole like that?" Asking those questions, coping with your anger, leads to personal growth and maturation.

Now what if instead you come home and light a joint—or these days a blunt—smoke some weed and think to yourself "f__ those a_holes!" You let the cannabis calm you down, and you're at peace. But now you have bypassed the opportunity for personal growth.

I have seen many people who have suffered severe recurrent trauma in childhood. Those who did not indulge in substances generally learned to deal with their past well enough to function in life. Like Holocaust survivors, they suffer on the inside, but they do function. People who suffered abuse in childhood and turned to substances for solace, generally cannot function without those substances. They call it "self-medicating."

To return to our primary population—those who did not particularly suffer in childhood—we still find them unprepared for the rigors of adulthood. As adolescents on the inside, they are unable to handle the demands laid on grownups. They become "depressed" and obnoxious without their substances. They remain exquisitely sensitive to events: inordinately unhappy when things don't go their way, inordinately happy when things go right. They have never learned to cope with adversity or to keep their happiness in bounds. Add to that the unmodulated hyperactivity of ADHD, and you can see how clinicians mistake what they see for "bipolar disorder."

Here is your first opportunity to refrain from doing harm: antipsychotics—especially when given to nonpsychotic people—can have serious long-term deleterious medical consequences. Psychiatrically, they have been shown to worsen a person's emotional stability in adulthood when they are used in childhood. Anticonvulsants often carry the risk of dangerous side effects. Just as importantly, artificially dampening an inmate's emotional responses is depriving him (or her) the opportunity to grow, to begin to master his or her responses to the slings and arrows of outrageous fortune. You may think you are doing a kindness to prescribe a "medication" (actually a drug) to help an inmate sleep. But this is a tendency he has had all of his life. No medication will help him sleep for the rest of his life. Every sleeping pill stops working. The best thing you can do for someone with ADHD insomnia is to let him find his own path, whether it is learning how to rest or learning to work 2-1/2 jobs to stay busy while he is awake or getting treatment for his ADHD. These are life skills, and drug "help" just puts off the learning of these necessary skills.

Traumatized as Children

The next group of inmates seeking care I have already alluded to: people who have taken psychological hits when they were young. If you ask every single person you see about traumas suffered in childhood, you will discover how pervasive such a history is in the population of people who seek psychiatric care. It is no different at the jailhouse.

Make no mistake; we are not talking about people whose mothers favored the other children. We are talking about preschoolers who were left on their own for days at a time; children who watched their mother's boyfriends beating her so badly they feared for her life; children who were beaten because they were hyperactive or just looked like their biological fathers; children who were molested or raped and told they deserved it or they wanted it. Such people have persistent nightmares and intrusive thoughts of these traumas. They may be afraid to go to sleep at night and don't know why. They were molested at night but they don't connect their fear of the night with their old anticipation of abuse. And often if they do not show classic signs of PTSD, you can still see a clear change in the trajectories of their lives.

They often have borderline personality disorders. Not infrequently they hear voices. And sadly, if they pull through with enough functional ability to volunteer for one of the armed services, their set of experiences in childhood puts them at greater risk for PTSD when they are exposed to war trauma. A colleague recalled an excellent metaphor for this: the cracked vessel. Consider the childhood trauma to be the cracks in the vessel. A vessel with cracks in it does not stand up well to pressure and when it is stressed it falls apart. We see many such cracked vessels in our jailhouse practice.

Although this traumatized group of people will have moods they can hardly control, they do not have bipolar disorder. In fact, whatever comfort they can obtain from any medication or drug can only be temporary: our medications work on the head; their suffering is in the heart. They need psychotherapy, not pills.

Another aspect of this group is how they are mistreated by mental health professionals. Mental health professionals often do not inquire into past histories. Instead they tend to blow off adverse childhood experiences. They in essence belittle these sad people, saying their back-grounds do not count; they call them "bipolar" or say they have "character disorders." In a way, this is simply further abuse.

Worse, recent research indicates that if such people are "treated" with antipsychotics, as those with "bipolar disorder" often are, they have worse outcomes as adults, suffering from "bipolar spectrum" and other such maladies (actually dysthymia).

Finally, we have to deal with the fact that the DSM's and the ICD's do not fully capture adverse childhood experiences (ACE's). There isn't good nomenclature for it. These people often do not show a classic PTSD syndrome, so "Chronic PTSD" doesn't really describe it; nor does "Dysthymia." In the mental health field, we need a name or set of names to describe the adverse experiences of children.

Substance Abusers

The third important group of people we must understand is the group of substance abusers: the alcoholics, the potheads, the cokeheads and dope fiends, the benzodiazepine-dependent, the quetiapine addicts. They may or may not have additional issues like ADHD, PTSD and borderline personality disorder. But they are *not* "self-medicating."

The whole idea of excusing drug use as "self-medication" is psychiatry's greatest act of enabling substance abusers. The concept is permission-giving for criminal behavior and such concepts as 'addiction substitutes.' Drinking and/or using drugs is all about getting high. It might also be a way of avoiding bad feelings, of hiding from one's troubles—but it is not any kind of medication. In fact, even some medications are drugs and some medicines used for side effects are drugs. It is no accident that drug addicts, alcoholics and people with ADHD and BPD ask for benzodiazepines, doxepin, chlorpromazine, diphenhydramine, gabapentin, hydroxyzine, mirtazapine, quetiapine and trazodone: they simply do not want to experience life raw. They want drugs to cover their experiences so they don't feel them. But it is most important that they do so.

People who are suddenly bereft of their substances typically go through a three-phase process: the acute withdrawal or "kicking" phase, nominally a week; the middle-term classic detox phase, typically a month or so; the rehabilitation phase, nominally a year, when their moods go up and down as they re-learn or learn the rudiments of emotional self-modulation. Note that recent research documents that craving continues to be an issue during this phase. And people who work in rehab talk of PAWS (post-acute withdrawal syndrome).

As such, jail environments can be some of the best detox facilities imaginable: if an inmate "just can't stand it anymore" and wants to go out and get high to relieve his stress . . . he cannot do so. So the addict goes through a number of crises of the spirit and he learns that having feelings will not kill him. This is powerful knowledge, and enables personal growth. If you take these painful feelings from him you deny him those growth experiences, and he leaves jail or prison unchanged, ready to relapse and bound to fail; to return to jail.

On the other hand, people who have been forced to actually experience their feelings come through stronger. I have been told by many an inmate, "Jail saved my life." Given their histories—given their alcohol, drug and medicine histories—they are not exaggerating.

Sleep

A lot of inmates spend their lives "running the streets." They tend to be up at night and sleep during the day. They have a different diurnal rhythm from most of us. The key to changing their sleep-wake cycle is through something called sleep hygiene. This involves getting up every morning for weeks—maybe months—and going to bed at the same time every night. What is interesting is that when CO's or nurses check on these inmates, the inmates are usually sound asleep

Traumatized in Adolescence or Adulthood

There is another important group: those who have had trauma in adolescence and adulthood. This often happens to people who were traumatized as children but it also happens to people without a problematic background. Examples include rape victims, veterans of war, victims of domestic violence, victims of criminal gangs, victims of crime generally and survivors of motor vehicle accidents. They may even be victims of violence by the police. If the trauma was bad enough, the victim may hear voices. Treating such a person for schizophrenia does not reach the trauma and adds the risk of diabetes and obesity to lives already fraught with trouble.

Summary

Understanding these groups is essential to practicing psychiatry in jails and prisons. Those imprisoned will come to you asking for soporific medications for sleep. They want drugs to calm down. If you prescribe comfort pills, you will be harming them over the long term, not helping them.

First of all, do no harm.

(In first three editions of this book, "Street Talk for Shrinks" was here. That section is now in Appendix G—Glossary.)

Chapter 3
Treatment Philosophy

Doctors from earliest times have been in business of relieving suffering due to disease. That is our calling. We look at the short term and long term benefits to our patients. As physicians that is our intention. As psychiatrists we treat mental illnesses. That is our job. If you are a nurse practitioner, an advanced practice nurse or a PA, that is your job too.

In our private practices we are used to dealing with patients who come to us honestly describing their suffering. For the most part they are not dependent on substances and they have no reason to lie about their symptoms. These assumptions are not valid for the population we see in jails. Inmates often lie to get drugs or to obtain a favorable report: they believe that our observations are used in court, which is not true. In essence, we are not there to please inmates. We are there to treat their mental illnesses.

If suffering due to illness is a river, we physicians trace the tributaries to the sources of suffering and endeavor to stop them up, one by one. If we are successful. the river of suffering will dry up. If the patient (the word derives from Latin 'sufferer') contributes to his or her own suffering, we can either convince him to change his ways or accept that some trickle of suffering will get through, no matter what we do.

Nurses, on the other hand, have traditionally embraced the whole patient and all her suffering, no matter the source. While nurses often help doctors in their search for the sources of suffering, nurses have not been called to address sources of discomfort, but to comfort patients. When you transition from the traditional nursing role to nurse practitioner, you transition from nursing to the medical profession. Whatever you call yourself, you are a doctor in the eyes of the patient. You too get to search for the sources of suffering. Welcome to the club.

As doctors it is *not* always our job to prescribe something the inmate wants. As physicians it is our job to prescribe what the inmate needs. The commonest example is the inmate who wants "something for pain." While the complaint may be the truth or may be a lie, the inmate is usually fishing for opiates. If the inmate gets those opiates he may never have to deal with his circumstances because he feels so "good." As we have seen, the use of drugs impairs the maturation process. This 'substitute addiction' model for substance users (think benzodiazepines for the alcoholic, methadone for the heroin addict) leaves them still addicted. But now they are dependent not only on substances but dependent on the medical profession as well. Under this model, we become their drug dealers.

There is a tradition in medicine called "Loeb's Laws of Medicine." They are attributed to Robert

F. Loeb MD, a famous internist who flourished in the middle of the twentieth century and who co-authored the Cecil-Loeb textbook of medicine. These "laws" have been variously formulated. My first intern—due in a week to be a resident—told them to us as follows:

- First of all, do no harm.
- Secondly: if what you're doing works, keep doing it.
- Thirdly: if what you're doing doesn't work, stop doing it.
- Fourthly: above all, never let your patient fall into the hands of a surgeon.

The fourth item was a joke but a pointed joke. The intern explained that Loeb, an internist, was in competition with surgeons. Also, surgery was fairly barbaric a long time ago. This leads to an alternate formulation of the fourth law:

- Never make the treatment worse than the disease.

In psychiatry that last has been a close call.

You will find that the principles—enunciated in Loeb's Laws—permeate the approach to doing psychiatry in jails.

The Source of the Traditional Psychiatric Model

As psychiatrist we are used to dealing with chronic schizophrenics. These people need our help. Because they experience delusions and hallucinations, they need our medicines to keep the demons at bay. Because they lack spontaneity and have other disabilities of executive function (they don't pay attention to the significance of a date, for example) they need us and our colleagues to help them make their way in this complicated unhelpful world. While this may work for schizophrenics, this is not a model we should carry to the jailhouse.

(Aside: Even patients are beginning to kick back at this dependency model. Note the rise of 'consumers' and the recovery movement.)

(Another aside: The treatments we proffer to patients often seem to violate the alternate fourth law 'Never make the treatment worse than the disease.' If schizophrenia is worse than first-generation antipsychotics, then the illness must be very bad indeed.)

Our task at the jailhouse is to help inmates get back on their feet. We treat the mental illnesses they have, but we need to foster an attitude that they are independent, capable human beings. Neither they nor we should think of them as dependent on the medical profession. It may be that an inmate recovers from her depression; or he was crashing and never needed the medicine in the first place, especially since he has adjusted to jail now. Such an inmate may abandon active psychiatric treatment. Good.

Jail is a stressful place. For someone with substance issues, a jail is a place where she can no longer get her substances. First, there is the withdrawal when the body is screaming for its lost substances. Then there is the classic detoxification phase, when the mind is screaming for its lost substances. Then there is the rehabilitation phase, when the addict living his life is screaming for his missing substances; a person must learn to cope with the world without substances. Often this is stressful *per se,* since the substance user has not developed the coping skills needed for responsible adult behavior, much less parenting.

Even for people without substance dependence, jail is a stressful place. An inmate is stripped of her usual clothes and much of her jewelry. The cell phone is taken (woe be to she who wants to make a phone call and cannot remember the number; the phone with the numbers on it is in lockup). The place may be strange. It is noisy—the other inmates seem to make a lot of noise. She may feel anxious, tense. She cannot sleep at night. She is worried about her life on the outside. And these are the normal responses.

We do not treat normal responses. We treat mental illness.

We do not treat normal responses. We treat mental illness.

We do not treat normal responses. We treat mental illness.

There. I said it three times. It must be true.

Inmates often come to us asking for drugs to treat their normal responses to incarceration. They ask us for drugs to treat their upsetness at their last conversation with their significant other, with their distress over the fact that a loved one is ill or dying or in some kind of trouble. They would like a benzodiazepine, or some amitriptyline, chlorpromazine, doxepin, diphenhydramine, trazodone, hydroxyzine, mirtazapine, quetiapine, anything to take the edge off their distress. But think about it a second. Do you take a pill when you or your loved one is in trouble? Or do you cope?

The philosophy of the pill-taker, of the person who believes that in facing life stressors she deserves "a little something to get by" is fundamentally a drug-abuser's mindset. People used to talk about "lying awake all night worrying" about something. No more. Now the people who might have lain awake worrying are expected to take a pill and go to sleep. In essence, no one is expected to handle bad news, but to take a pill and not deal with it. This is the mindset we are combatting.

So to be clear, we do not treat "anxiety" (this cannot be taken at face value; look at Chapter 5 and Appendix G). We do not treat insomnia. We do not treat ADHD, since so many inmates have this "disorder" that we would end up treating the great majority of inmates, and with abusable substances. (The exception is when the ADHD is so bad that the CO's are complaining about the inmate's behavior. And even then you don't use stimulants with adults.) We treat legitimate mental illnesses—the psychoses, depression, mania, PTSD, etc.

We treat mental illnesses with medications, not drugs.

Drugs vs Medications

When inmates complain of depression, treat them with citalopram, fluoxetine, sertraline or some other SSRI. If they truly have an anxious depression one of the SSRI's or an SNRI like venlafaxine or duloxetine will help them. Or you can treat with an SSRI combined with buspirone. But if they were only drug seeking, they will lose interest in the treatment process, stop taking their meds and not come for follow-up. That is one less inmate you will have on your roster. You will have more room for inmates with true psychiatric disorders.

This then is your non-traditional model for psychiatry in jails:

We do not treat normal responses. We treat mental illnesses.

Inmates Talk About You

Inmates talk about you. They share stories about your interactions and prescribing practices. They make up histories to appeal to you. If they don't make up histories they change them to better fit your prescribing practices. If you never prescribe desirable drugs, you would think that it won't matter what inmates say. But think again. Inmates will lie to get antipsychotics, because those antipsychotics can have desirable sedating side effects. Make sure when you prescribe them, that an inmate is truly psychotic.

A few miscellaneous comments:

Always use meds for on-label purposes. Gabapentin and topiramate, for example, are anticonvulsants that have been studied in psychiatric illness—and have failed whenever they were studied. They have earned no FDA indications for psychiatric illnesses. Thus they are "off-label" for all psychiatric conditions. The fact that people still take them suggests of course that they can be used as drugs. After all, gabapentin targets the same GABA receptor that the benzodiazepines do (see appendix ME under gabapentin). And topiramate calms you down. So psychiatrists in jails do not prescribe these medications. They are only prescribed by physical medical practitioners for seizures, neuropathic pain and migraine.

Always start with a single med for a single condition. A schizophrenic, for example, might do quite well on risperidone alone. Someone with depression may do well with citalopram alone.

Inmates are comfortable with being dependent on their psychiatrist. This is a comfortable, familiar role. In the inmate's mind, the psychiatrist is replacing the drug dealer. In fact, the roles are equivalent, with the inmate turning to the drug dealer when he cannot get in to see the psychiatrist. That just reinforces the "self-medicating" concept. The sole advantage you have over the drug dealer is that your meds are legal, where his are illegal.

Think about it a minute. Are you comfortable with being an inconvenient drug dealer?

Philosophy of Treatment

(5/16/09) [original trade names replaced with generic names]

The following is a brief summary of jail psychiatry as of 2009. I was writing instructions for a psychiatrist coming from office practice to substitute for me. It was handwritten, done in a hurry, as a single draft. I have crossed through parts that no longer apply:

"**Basic Principles:**
1.   We do not treat insomnia
2.   We do not treat anxiety.
3.   Psychiatrists do not treat withdrawal.
4.   Psychiatrists do not treat seizures, or other medical conditions.
5.   We never, ever prescribe benzodiazepines for any reason whatsoever.
6.   We do not treat ADD/ADHD.
7.   We never ever prescribe stimulants.

8.   If the hyperactivity component of ADHD is causing discipline problems, try clonidine, lithium, and/or [chlorpromazine] or [bupropion].[Note that as a soporific, chlorpromazine is no longer used in jails; because bupropion is often abused, it is used less often in jails]

9.   For depression, use an SSRI first; it's not going to have desirable side effects. NOTE that [mirtazapine], trazodone and [amitriptyline] are non-formulary.

10.   NO [quetiapine]. The addicts know it and love it as a heroin-enabler. It is not a legitimate drug for "bipolar disorder." Generally, the dose starts low, helps for a while, then, must be repeatedly increased. Finally, there is a withdrawal syndrome. [quetiapine] is heroin in a pill, not a medication.

11.   I have one patient who takes [quetiapine] for schizophrenia—all other meds have failed and we know this case very well.

12.   Do not over-diagnose bipolar disorder. Too many people have that diagnosis applied when their moods range from normal happiness to very unhappy. This is dysthymia, not bipolar disorder.

13.   People complain of "racing thoughts." Generally this is anxiety and real-world worries that should keep them up at night. Worrying about your circumstances is normal. Trying to medicate normal worries away is to act like a drug dealer, not a doctor.

14.   Many people are restless, can't sleep, anxious, can't stop thinking. They had ADHD as

children and still have it. Drugs and alcohol seem to prevent the hyperactivity component from fading. This is not bipolar disorder.

15.   Adults may appear silly, speeded up, even euphoric when things are going well, then plunge to dysphoric depths when things go wrong.

16.   Think twelve-year-olds.

17.   These are people who started using young and never grew up. They have adult bodies and adolescent minds. They are not bipolar.

18.   Think 12-year-old ADHD kids and see what you get. Again, not bipolar.

19.   In summary, unless you know for a fact that someone has been manic, don't buy "bipolar disorder" in this population.

20.   PTSD. I always ask about history of parental alcoholism, drug addiction and violence; bad things happening in childhood—beaten, abused, neglected, molested, seen people killed—and military history.

21.   PTSD is big in this population. Among those who have been abused, you see many "panic attacks" and "OCD" as conversion symptoms—ways to avoid flashbacks and intrusive thoughts. I teach inmates to understand that their brain is trying to teach them something, or warn them. If they can visualize that younger self, they can observe the flashback, or intrusive thought. The key: the earlier self feared dying, but did not die. This is what the current inmate knows that the earlier self did not.

22.   Voices. Not all voices are hallucinations. In this population, most voices are not hallucinat-

ions.   Hallucinations are false sensory perceptions. Most people here have intrapsychic voices,
generally due to PTSD. For drug-abuse-related
hallucinations,   [chlorpromazine]   [deprecated
today] is best. Before using any new generation
antipsychotic, try an old one. The old meds work
fine."

I would tweak a few points in the above list,
but it was a decent beginning. See the Afterword
for the updated version.

Chapter 4
Getting a History
& Mental Status

Throughout the history of medicine, all medical diagnoses and treatment has begun with getting a history. Psychiatry is no different. Unless you get a good history—one that addresses the pertinent points—your diagnosis is likely to be partly or wholly incorrect.

A pertinent history need not take long. These days I can do a typical assessment in 20 minutes or less. In what follows I will give the questions I ask, then explain why I ask those questions in the manner I do. After that, we will cover some answers from inmates and what they mean. Always keep in mind that an inmate may be lying to you, so try as much as possible to ask open-ended questions. No sense in showing the inmate how to lie to you and how to fake her way into getting meds for a nonexistent illness.

You were probably taught to ask patients about their histories subject by subject. I have tried that, but abandoned it in favor of a chronological approach. This chronological approach assures that I will miss nothing important to the inmate.

Also, you were probably taught to ask about symptoms in a doctor-centered way. You must ask about symptoms as inmates experience them.

Demographics

Important information will include an inmate's age, his legal marital status, his date of commitment and whether he was on some sort of withdrawal protocol. You will have to ask about marital status and children:

Married/single/separated/divorced/widowed? Children?

A sample handwritten entry might read "41yo SepWM DOC [date of commitment] 12/1/17 on [chlordiazepoxide] w/d prot for opiates and etoh." It may be cryptic (an EMR version may have the abbreviations explicated, as noted later) but it quickly tells the medical reader whether the inmate was a recent commit still in withdrawal or detox, or is someone who has had ample time to develop a depression or an adjustment disorder in response to his incarceration. The inmate's having children may have a bearing on what they have to live for (suicidality).

Reason for Referral / Chief Complaint

Begin with the reason for the referral. This information you get from referrers. Did the inmate tell them he had a history of psychiatric treatment? Current psych meds? Feeling suicidal? Was she acting strangely? Looking depressed? This material sets the stage.

Next comes the traditional beginning of a medical workup—the Chief Complaint. I will typically begin:

Hi. I'm Dr. Hume, the psychiatrist here. How can I help you? or *Why are you seeing a psychiatrist today?*

Often the inmate will say "I'm not getting my meds" or "I'm bipolar."

I'll write that down but then I'll say

I'd like to know what's bothering you right now.

I don't care that some other psychiatrist called the inmate "bipolar." These days everybody is called "bipolar." You'd think there was a plague of it out there, despite a stable prevalence of about 2% of the population.

Likewise, although it is interesting to know that an inmate wants his "meds" (usually they are legally prescribed drugs), his statement of current complaints can be highly illuminating. Someone who is stable on her antidepressants for, example, will usually have no complaints, but believes that she will need to restart her meds to keep from relapsing. If an inmate has been taking drugs, on the other hand, he will be frantic to get on something to replace them; so he will tell you he was taking trazodone or clonazepam or quetiapine, depending on what he believes you can prescribe him.

If a man has been in jail more than a month and tells you he is unmotivated and without energy, sad and irritable, "stressing" and "lashing out" you start to think about depression. In any case, the chief complaint is a thumbnail capsule of a person's distress. It is the door to what ails the patient.

Past History

Next we get into the background history. Although some people put the HPI—History of the Present Illness—first, I find that without a background, the HPI can be misleading. Often you end up getting the history twice. Start with the background, and start that at the beginning. The more research is done, the clearer it is that adverse events suffered in childhood have enduring deleterious effects in adulthood, from depression to diabetes. There is even an acronym, ACE—adverse childhood experiences—to cover the subject.

4 – Getting a History and Mental Status

Where were you born and raised? [State]?

Here I will add the state as part of the question. The reason I add it came from a peculiarity I noticed in New Jersey. Rather than tell you they came from around Newark (a suburb of New York City) or the Pine Barrens (home to Ft. Dix/McGuire Air Force Base) they will tell you the little tiny town they grew up in, as if it mattered. Supplying the state tells them the scope of your question. You will find the occasional person who was born in Germany where his father was stationed; or in Mexico. You won't know unless you ask.

Some people were raised nearby; others "all over." When someone was raised "all over" his father might have been in the military. Or was a drunk who couldn't keep a job. Or the mother went with one man or the other. You begin to get some notion of the stability in the inmate's upbringing—or the lack thereof.

Who raised you?

I love it when inmates tell me they raised themselves. I get to tell them "You didn't raise yourself when you were one."

Who took care of you?

I'm particularly interested in children being handed off. For example, an inmate was raised by her maternal great-grandmother until she was 12 years old; and then by her maternal grandmother. Or someone was taken from the mother and placed in foster care.

If the inmate responds "My parents" I ask

Your biological parents? Together?

Sometimes an inmate's parents ping-ponged him between households. Sometimes they were together until they split when the inmate was *x* years old. Sometimes "my parents" means "my mother and my stepfather." The point is that "my parents" is a phrase that means different things to different people. If you make assumptions, you can lose potentially valuable information.

Was your mother an alcoholic or a drug addict?
Your stepfather ... ?
Your biological father ... ?

An inmate may answer "They're deceased." I respond

When you were a kid

In part, I want to know for genetic reasons. Based on careful research done in Scandinavia we know that the biological children of alcoholics are more prone to depression, for example, even when they are raised by genetically unrelated nonalcoholic adoptive parents. And if someone is raised by an alcoholic or an addict there are always consequences. Many inmates you see are ACOA (Adult Child of Alcoholics) or the equivalent children of drug addicts. For the latter be wary of the addict-mother's peddling their "services" for drugs.

Just remember that a parent cannot be kid-centered when she is substance-centered.

If the mother was an alcoholic or drug addict when the inmate was young, we must ask him if his mother was drinking when she was pregnant with him. Or whether she was using. Recent information has been emerging about fetal alcohol spectrum disorders and prenatal exposure to alcohol and drugs. Since these conditions mimic the emotional dysregulation seen in BPD and are often characterized by irritability, they can be mistaken for bipolar disorder. Proper documentation of an inmate's history can help your diagnosis if you have cause to reconsider the case as more information emerges. The better our diagnoses, the better the treatment we offer.

Did anybody beat you when you were young?
Did anybody molest you when you were young?
Was anybody verbally abusive to you?

Here we hit the trauma history head on. We get the history of abuse early because abuse can start early in a person's life. Some people were beaten for discipline. The inmate sees it was for discipline and may even think it was deserved (kids with ADHD, for example, typically get in lots of trouble in our urban society and often receive beatings as a result.). But a beating is a beating and sets the inmate up to be more violent to others in turn.

Beating "for no reason" is generally worse; the boy who has his head bashed through a wall by an enraged drunken stepfather; a child who is thrown down a flight of stairs. These are frightening events, fraught with the experience of total loss of control.

Molestation is of course complicated. Generally I want to know the ages at which a patient was molested—sexual violation as a preschooler versus violation at an elementary school age versus violation as an adolescent. These have very different consequences for the development of a person. Also, what was the degree of relationship between the molester and the victim? Was the molester a babysitter? Male or female? Was it a man in the neighborhood? A foster brother? A coach? A stepfather? The boyfriend of a mother? Dad's drinking buddy? All of these details matter. The effects are outside the scope of a discussion on history but as jail clinicians, we need to understand the overall dimensions of an inmate's experience of sexual abuse. Depending on the inmate, you may ask more about trauma. Sometimes you won't ask these questions, but you will always keep them in the back of your head, just in case.

Finally, ask if the inmate told someone at the time. It is one thing to tell a sib. But what if a child tells her mother that the mother's boyfriend's son is molesting her, and the mother calls her a liar? What if she tells her mother that the mother's boyfriend is molesting her, but the mother not only does nothing but continues to live with the man? What is the child to think? How should she feel? Some victims are cowed; some unremittingly angry. In any case, such events just might have a wee bit to do with the victim's subsequent growth and development. Just a wee bit.

Did anything terrible happen when you were young? Did you see anybody killed when you were young?
Did your father beat your mother?
Did you see someone else getting abused?

The experience of watching your mother get beaten, scared to death she will be killed, and helpless to do anything, is profoundly traumatizing. As an inmate becomes older, he might have tried to intervene and been beaten because of it. The inmate will often spontaneously tell you about these dramatic events. Recently, for example, an inmate told of going in and out of foster care and extended family situations. He would see his sibs abused, commenting now, "I was too weak to protect them." What could a seven-year-old have done? But it says something about the sense of responsibility a child can feel and an intimation of the sense of failure that can pervade a case.

It may or may not surprise you to learn how many inmates have seen people shot, stabbed and killed. Sometimes it was someone close. Often they feared death themselves. And if Child and Youth removed a child from the home of an unfit mother? The child may have been traumatized by the removal and placement with a foster family, no matter how nice they were.

Do you get nightmares about those experiences?

Some inmates will say "I used to." Some say they still have nightmares and flashbacks though usually an inmate means an intrusive thought or memory and not an actual re-experiencing of the event. Of course we are fishing for PTSD here. The questions are perforce leading questions, unless they were part of the chief complaint. But sometimes these explorations lead to an explanation of symptoms (see below re- hallucinations). Often victims do not have a classic picture of PTSD, but you can see how the trauma(s) affected their lives.

Did you have a hard time sitting still and paying attention?

If the inmate answers yes to those screening questions I ask more about ADHD. Otherwise I move on. We have a lot of ground to cover in a short time.

Did you have a hard time getting to sleep at night from racing thoughts?
Were you impulsive? Did you do things suddenly on the spur of the moment, not thinking about them first?

OK—direct questions again. But these are questions we need to know the answers to and asking open-ended questions about ADHD symptoms is too time-consuming. Generally people who were not troubled with these problems will say so.

I used to ask a number of questions before I settled on the above four screening questions. I asked about mind wandering; I asked about memory: someone who is not paying attention will not form a memory. I learned that most inmates do not know the difference between impulsive and compulsive behavior unless I concretely ask about doing things without forethought.

With a past history of neglect, there are times when positive ADHD questions look more like depression than ADHD. If you compound a low IQ with depression you can get answers that mimic ADHD. Basically you must use your overall feel for a case to get this one right.

Did you get angry easily and hit people?
Did you get in a lot of fights?

I don't often ask about this, but sometimes the question needs to be asked. Often inmates will say "I got p___d off easy but I hit walls, not people." Inmates whose upbringing included violence will often do violence to others. When people have expressions of anger or violence that are more than what you would expect from the provocation, the question of Intermittent Explosive Disorder (IED) arises. This leaves a question the condition: Is IED a biological disorder? Or does it express the sum of a person's experiences so that he will not resist an urge to do violence? Since the question is open in the literature I try to be conservative: I will not diagnose IED unless someone comes from a nonviolent background and still does violence to others, with that tendency originating in childhood. You may diagnose this differently if at all. For example PED (prenatal exposure to drugs) or ND-PAE are possibilities. So is DMDD (F34.81).

Were you in special education, special classes? Behavior classes? Alternative schools? Did you get Ritalin, Adderall, Concerta? Did anyone tell your caregivers you needed meds? Did other kids make fun of you for being slow?

Often this inquiry merely confirms that other clinicians recognized the inmate's ADHD when he or she was in school.

Why are we interested in childhood ADHD? When kids grow up, they often still have their ADHD, and it leads them into trouble.

The last question is fishing for cognitive deficiency or intellectual disability (the current term for what used to be called mental retardation). Someone who is "slow" often lacks cognitive reserves for learning to cope with adverse circumstances or events. She might make poor decisions or be led to make poor decisions.

At this point the main part of the background history is complete. But if I have time I will ask about military service, mainly for high school graduates and men old enough to have been drafted.

Sometimes inmates allege PTSD symptoms resulting from military service. They complain about nightmares and flashbacks. Although you may not have served yourself, you can generally get a sense of whether the inmate is complaining about real symptoms or making it all up. It helps, of course, if the inmate knows in advance that you do not prescribe sedatives or hypnotics.

Did you try to enlist? Which branch?
When did you enlist? When did you get out? What was your highest rank?
What was your discharge rank? What kind of discharge did you receive?

A military service history can be done quickly. I will cover it in Appendix MI. However a person can be disqualified if he is not intelligent enough to pass the entrance exam. Or if he has a serious mental illness, he will not make it through basic training or boot camp. Often an illness like schizophrenia or bipolar disorder will have its onset during military service; the age of service corresponds to the peak age of onset for these disorders and the stress of military training will often provoke a manic episode or bring on a schizophreniform psychosis. These people are discharged.

Were you a loner? Did you hang out with friends?

Sometimes a person has the feel of being a schizophrenic (e.g.—showing Bleuler's 4 A's). Or he is complaining if psychotic symptoms now. When you have a situation like that, it is best to ask questions like this. Otherwise the questions go unasked.

Substance Use and Abuse

You can ask about substances (alcohol and drugs) now, before you get a PMH; or you can ask it after, before the HPI:

What substances did you use regularly, daily?

Although you can discern some patterns the selection of drugs does not correlate well with diagnosis. As a practical matter abuse of two substances requires two diagnoses; abuse of three or more qualifies as F19.2 (304.8) Polysubstance Dependence.

When did you start substances?

When the inmate used drugs steadily from adolescence it has a significant effect on their maturation process. If an inmate seems mature he probably had a long break in his substance abuse—prison, for instance.

If an inmate has been abstinent, for how long?

Be careful here. An inmate can tell you she was abstinent but she was taking a legally prescribed benzodiazepine or quetiapine or methadone. Yes, she was legal; but no, she was not clean and will not behave like a person who has been clean for long years.

Past Medical History (PMH)

The next part of the workup is the past medical history (PMH). Why get the PMH at this point? *Because we're doctors, after all.* We care— or should care—about the inmate's overall medical condition. In addition, the clinical orientation will help us get a more honest history of the inmate's substance use through a gradual transition. Finally some medical conditions produce psychiatric symptoms. But that's another section. For now, start with the question:

What are you allergic to?

This can be a surprisingly revealing question. Aside from the normal "allergy" to milk (usually lactose intolerance but occasionally a true allergy) the inmate may tell you he is "allergic" to Haldol or Thorazine. Of course by now you know enough to unpack that statement. Usually you get a description of acute dystonia, even akathisia. But sometimes you get a description of rashes or other indications of a true allergy. If an inmate describes side effects from extra-pyramidal system side effects (EPS SE's or simply EPS) to hyperprolactinemia, list the offending medication as a sensitivity. Note also that somebody gave this person an antipsychotic.

By 'allergies' we mean allergic reactions. Those are common enough. Keep in mind that a person is as likely to be allergic to a dye or other excipient as she is to be allergic to the medicine itself.

Do you have any medical problems—asthma, Hepatitis, HIV, head injuries, anemia, broken bones, high blood pressure, seizures?

Make your own list; then repeat it every time you see an inmate. The repetition will cause you to memorize it so you will not forget mentioning the main illnesses. These conditions will inform your psychiatric diagnoses.

Ever get hit on the head and knocked out, like in a wreck or a fight?

A large number of inmates have been in at least one motor vehicle accident (MVA), fights or an assault. The "knocked out" question is an interesting one. If not prefaced with the phrase "hit on the head" you can get someone telling you about general anesthesia.

Also ask about high blood pressure, diabetes, cancer—all the usual suspects. This is not really a Review of Systems as much as it is a Parade of Diseases. I am always surprised, for example, that I get a steady number of inmates who have a history of Crohn's disease. In any case having a general medical history will inform your decisionmaking. They may tell you about how they were shot (gunshot wound or GSW) and when, which will allow you start to differentiate between an anxiety disorder and PTSD.

A seizure history is important. It needs to be explored for a history of partial complex seizure symptoms and temporal lobe symptoms (hearing voices or music, smelling out-of-place smells, lots of deja-vu). Not that we are looking for an explanation of the inmate's crimes here; but a history of seizure-related symptoms suggests a possible intervention with anticonvulsants not associated with a "bipolar" disorder. That said, I have seen people with a non-convulsive temporal lobe dysfunction (TLD) who have had a near-complete remission of their problems with a small amount of carbamazepine.

Here we can include the fact of prenatal exposure to drugs (PED) or ND-PAE if you have not already covered this. Sometimes a lifelong seizure disorder can alert you to an inmate's cognitive impairment.

Psychiatric History (HPI)

Although a middle-class practice assumes that a person was essentially well and then became ill, you cannot make this assumption in jail. Most inmates come with the baggage of a rough childhood, a tortured adolescence and an adulthood marked by crime and/or domestic violence. For that reason you cannot get a History of the Present Illness (HPI) and assume that you have captured the essence of the inmate's illness. You will miss it most of the time.

Likewise, in cases of real psychiatric illness, you will not have time to do a detailed unpacking of the HPI. For one thing, because most inmates who come to see psychiatrists have long-term issues, the HPI is not as important as the inmate's background. But even when the HPI is important, the inmate often will not remember the details of her illness, but only the highlights. So we get what is important, or we are limited to what we can get.

How many times have you tried to kill yourself?

If the inmate wants to talk about when they thought about suicidal ideation make it clear that you care about whether they tried to do something about it—or not. Sometimes I will ask clarifying questions to separate actual attempts (suicidal acts done with the intent of dying) from gestures (parasuicidal acts done with the intent of producing an effect on someone else; terrorism, if you will). You might also ask about self-injury. If an inmate has never tried to kill herself she will say so. If the most recent attempt was . . . recent . . . you will want to know if the inmate was suicidal from a depression or from circumstances or both. You might have to be concerned about another attempt (or gesture) in jail.

How many times have you been an inpatient on a psych unit or in a mental hospital for psych?

By this you mean times that an inmate at least spent the night. A psych unit is where patients wear street clothes and walk around, not where they wear hospital gowns and stick to their beds. You are not interested in MICA, dual-diagnosis or rehab admissions here, just pure psych. I ask about both kinds of places because some people will tell you they have not been in a mental hospital when they have been an inpatient in a psychiatry unit and vice versa.

Why?

Now you find out if the inmate was hospitalized for suicidal ideation or something else. Sometimes the inmate will get vague about the reasons for admission. Sometimes he doesn't know. Vague reasons for admission to a psych unit suggest admissions for psychosis—schizophrenia or mania. Sometimes an inmate will tell you that he complained of suicidal ideation so that he could get some help for his substance issues.

Then we get into the meat of a mental illness. Sometimes an inmate was the victim of significant domestic violence by an abusive partner and has post-traumatic stress disorder symptoms. Or he might have nightmares and hypervigilance ever since he was shot. Or she has a depression that she has had since she was abused in childhood; but she was using drugs as a tool of emotion-avoidance and only experiences her feelings when she is off drugs.

(A note on nightmares: if the inmate complains about nightmares, find out if they are repeated recurrences of a specific event, or if they are on various subjects, even if they all have the same theme. The former are symptoms of a PTSD, where the latter are unconscious attempts to cope.)

When?

You will want to know when the inmate started going to hospital, and when he stopped. A boy who was in a psychiatric hospital as a child might have been there because of ADHD and/or DMDD. Someone who started going to psychiatric hospitals at 19 may have schizophrenia, bipolar disorder or BPD. Clues.

If you routinely ask about adverse events in childhood and adolescence and traumatic events in adulthood you will be shocked by how often our colleagues in the community ("on the street") have failed to ask about these. It is common to find people—especially urban dwellers—who have been exposed to trauma and diagnosed with "anxiety" or even "bipolar" disorder as if the trauma never occurred.

Some inmates are leading reasonably normal lives before they come to jail but life incarcerated begins to wear them down, making them feel depressed. These are people you see two months or more after their DOC (date of commitment).

Some inmates complain bitterly that they cannot sleep but somehow they cannot get up for morning meds because . . . (wait for it) . . . they are asleep. They have a dysfunctional sleep-wake cycle. They need counseling on sleep hygiene.

Some inmates are up all night touching things that belong to other inmates. Since touching what belongs to other inmates is risking a fight, this is a clue that the inmate in question might have a psychosis.

How do you feel when you're alone?

This is a key question in borderline personality disorder (BPD). Borderlines feel great emptiness, depending on others as anchors for their identities. This is especially pronounced when they are by themselves.

This is where your training in psychiatry kicks in, but be quick about it. Just as in a clinic, you do your assessment quickly.

Mental Status Examination (MSE)

The Mental Status Examination (MSE) is not properly part of a history at all, but it is something you have been accruing since the inmate walked into the waiting area.

Write down or type a mental status on every inmate you see. It is like the physical examination a GP writes when she sees you. It is part of a psychiatric encounter. Properly done, the entire interview is part of your mental status exam.

You should pay attention when an inmate enters the waiting area, even if you are engrossed in an interview with another inmate. Pay attention to the inmate's demeanor; how he moves, what he says. Then note the change as the inmate enters the interview area. Often the inmate transforms from a normal presentation to one of depression or a presentation with a collection of psychotic symptoms. But was the normalcy put on, with the inmate exposing his "real" self to you, the psychiatrist? Or is he faking his symptoms and he did not think you'd catch his being normal in the waiting area? You must decide, based on your full interview with the inmate.

Every school teaches a different mental status organization; but they all cover the same areas. Consider the following MSE as a guide only:

Appearance and Behavior Whether the inmate is alert, drowsy, agitated etc. Note if the inmate sits restlessly, jiggles her feet, bounces his leg but is otherwise normoactive vs hypoactive, psychomotor accelerated etc. Whether the inmate sits stiffly or leans forward on the doctor's desk, invading the interviewer's space or showing undue familiarity. If the inmate is responding to hallucinations (responding to internal stimuli—RIS) you may wish to include it here.

Mood and Affect Is the inmate happy, sad, scared or mad, or does he have a neutral mood?

Is he euthymic or anxious or angry? Then there is the affect. This is a wide-ranging topic that is important in transferring information about someone.

A person might superficially respond to social cues but not have the *broad* affect you see in normal people. Note that a broad affect indicates a suppleness in emotional responses with the inmate ranging into positive territory; a *normally responsive* affect lacks that excursion to positive feelings but the person otherwise responds normally to the emotional content of what is being discussed. But to have a normally responsive or broad affect the inmate must relate to you in a personal way, show a normal demeanor.

A person with schizophrenia may have a *blunted* affect but almost as often you will see someone with a *bland* affect—not fully responsive but not really blunted either; the person will be autistic, according to Bleuler; a *congruent* or socially responsive or *superficial* affect is almost like this. A person with a *dull* affect is generally lacking in intellectual capacity while someone with a *subdued* affect is responding normally but her responses are muted. This is the affect you sometimes see in a depressed person, or someone who is grieving, or fishing for sympathy or pretending to be depressed.

Does the person smile and laugh spontaneously and appropriately? If so note it. This points to an adjustment reaction or grief, rather than a major depression.

Demeanor Following mood and affect you will do well to comment on an inmate's demeanor. Is she childlike? Is he timid? Tearful? He may be polite—or obsequious. The range of human interaction is seemingly infinite. You need to comment on it. If he is selling his story, say so.

When you are dealing with psychiatric patients outside the jail, you most often see a guarded demeanor in paranoids. In jails, you see a guarded demeanor in malingerers as well as paranoids. Malingerers are trying to hide their normalcy, and paranoids are trying to hide themselves.

Flow of Thought A normal flow of thought is non-pressured, goal-directed, relevant and logical in association. Someone who talks rapidly but pauses to listen to you can have his speech described as *rushed,* but not pressured. Someone who puts in too many details can be described as *circumstantial,* but you may wish to reserve this description for conditions more pathological than narcissism or borderline personality, saying instead *highly detailed.* Some inmates who are lying, for example, may put in too much detail in their histories to persuade you how ill they are. Someone with a formal thought disorder may have pressured speech with irrelevant answers or tangentiality, flight of ideas, blocking etc.

Thought Content Here you will wish to note what was not present in order to cover yourself.

Note any *delusions* elicited or note that no delusions were elicited.

What comes up next are what I call Dr. Hume's Five Questions:

*Do you want to live or die?**

Sometimes people who do not want to kill themselves nonetheless want to die; the answer to this question can help you decide whom you need to help and how. If an inmate wants to live, note it. Such people usually will not try to kill themselves unless something happens after you see them. Having children often makes a difference here.

*Who do you want to kill?**

If the inmate replies "nobody" he has denied homicidal ideation.

*What are the voices saying right this second?**

Note that the form of this question often tangles up people who are not hallucinating; but this will ambush some psychotic people.

*Do you want to kill yourself right now?**

Some inmates will tell you that you have asked that question twice. But the question on wanting to live is future oriented, where the question on suicidal ideation is about an inmate's present wishes.

(* - These questions often provoke an inmate into laughing spontaneously and appropriately, so their very baldness helps your overall MSE.)

What is today's date?

Allow an inmate to guess. He may be oriented to the month and year. You are looking for dementia here—or vorbeireden. This question is properly part of the sensorium but it is part of the five questions I ask all inmates.

Sensorium Many inmates try not to remember the date—they seem to think that it makes the days go faster. If such an inmate thinks he does not know the date ask *What year is it?* followed by *What month is it?* followed by *Are we in early, middle or late [month]?* As you ask the inmate the date, it is clear that he is either in tune with his environment or not paying attention because he is delirious or attending to hallucinations. If an inmate is truly disoriented, you might be dealing with a delirium or a dementia. If he has the orientation within a few days he is fully oriented.

Memory People with schizophrenia often have a reasonably clear recollection up through the time they became ill; their memory for subsequent events tends to be vague, but they remember the most recent events pretty well. People with dementia, on the other hand, tend to recall past events but tend to have difficulty with immediate recall. People with ADHD tend to have difficulty with details in the past and recently unless they find the subject interesting—that material they tend to remember in detail. People who have had manic episodes might not remember being manic, or have a distorted memory of those events. These are common patterns of memory dysfunction; you do not so much as ask memory items as simply pay attention as you inquire about the history. The inmate's ability to recall her history tells you what you need to know about her memory. Conversely there may be intrusions of delusions or confabulations in an inmate's memory. They might even be lying.

Intellectual Functioning Some people never fully develop a normal cognitive ability. DSM-IV and earlier used 'mental retardation' for this condition. The official term by Federal statute is now 'intellectual disability.' Regardless of what you call it people suffering from this disability have less cognitive reserve for solving problems. Do not neglect this in formulating your diagnosis. Other problems with intellectual functioning include a psychotic process distorting cognitive function, impairment by delirium and so forth.

Most people's intellectual capacity is approximately average or within normal limits. Their intellects show no gross impairment. A psychotic person's intellectual functioning may be compromised by delusion or thought disorder. If a person's capacity and functioning diverge they may require commenting on this.

Insight and Judgment Usually these are lumped together but occasionally they deserve separate comment. When I&J deserve separate comments comment on them separately. For most inmates, Insight and Judgment are only fair; after all, they are in jail.

A **normal mental status** (a handwritten example): Alert, normoactive. Euthymic mood w/broad affect. Smiles&laughs spont&approp. FOT WNL. ō delusions. ō RIS. Wants to live. Denies HI, voices, SI. Ox3. Mem grossly intact. Intel fx WNL. I&J fair.

See? You can really boil it down.

Overall in gathering a history or assembling a mental status, quote the inmate liberally. For instance, an inmate came in. Smiling broadly he greeted the interviewer, asking "So when am I going to get drugs?" He could not better have encapsulated why we prescribed him nothing. We quoted him exactly.

Chapter 5
Diagnosing Inmates

In Chapter 2, we covered our main clinical populations. Now, how do we move from understanding people in general to understanding a particular inmate? Or at least how do we go about understanding what ails an inmate? We will explore diagnosis in this chapter. In general, the purpose of diagnosis is to communicate about patients; in particular, the purpose of diagnosis is to communicate about each particular inmate.

Luckily for us, we are allowed to make multiple diagnoses, since many of the inmates have multiple problems stacked on top of their lives—and that's before we even consider the stresses involved in getting arrested, living in jail, seeing affairs not taken care of, feeling one's life unraveling. But the latter are "simply" normal responses to the processes of incarceration and sequestration. As uncomfortable as they are, symptoms of these processes do not involve a mental illness. Since there is no mental illness involved, there is nothing for us to treat. We are not in the business of treating uncomfortable but normal responses to unfortunate events. We are not liquor stores or drug dealers—or we should not be. We are medical practitioners. Mental illness is hard enough.

Perhaps the most important considerations are motivation and prevarication. When inmates come to you complaining of depression or the like, have they been in jail for some months? Or have they recently been committed, and are having trouble coping with their circumstances? Or were they in withdrawal upon commitment and are now in detox? Maybe still in withdrawal? They may claim to have a mental illness, but are they telling the truth? Did the inmate last take psych meds when she was last in jail? Are you dealing with mental illness? Or is the inmate simply a "junkie" looking for you substitute stuff for his drugs? Or did something bad happen?

Diagnostic Classifications

You should familiarize yourself with ICD-10 and soon, ICD-11. You should bookmark the appropriate subdivisions of www.icd10data.com and use that reference frequently. You may never have it all memorized. Just remember that ICD-10, ICD-11 and their predecessor ICD-9 are billing codes, designed to classify illnesses for getting appropriate reimbursement for the care a doctor delivered. And recall that DSM stands for Diagnostic and Statistical Manual. The DSM's were designed to help researchers keep track of mental illnesses in the community. Neither reference is aimed at the busy clinician to help quickly parse the disorder (s)he faces. You can draw on those two resources, but in the end you must identify the diseases as you see them. Hopefully, what follows will help you.

The diagnoses which follow the format of a letter and a number are the ICD-10 code (psychiatric disorders are F-codes). In parentheses ( ) you will find the three-digit numbers of the ICD-9 codes that DSM-IV and DSM-5 follow; except DSM-5, too, has transitioned to ICD-10. Anticipating their use, the ICD-11 codes are enclosed in curly brackets {}.

An issue for some of you may be the specificity required by your payers. Hopefully, at the jail where you practice, specificity of diagnosis will not be required. Where you have a persnickety payer (you private practitioners will be nodding your heads) you will have to specify—sometimes beyond clinical—in detail. If you have such payers, do refer to www.icd10data.com on a regular basis. This is a small book, so diagnostic detail is not something we can cover here.

Externalizing

Inmates will frequently come to you telling you what others have diagnosed or observed. This is externalizing. Inmates do it a lot. They are attributing statements to others, so that later they can disavow those statements. It is a form of prevaricating—lying. In dealing with inmates, take what they have to say with a grain of salt. They tell you what they think you want to hear to provoke you into prescribing drugs for them. But when inmates are externalizing or triangulating, be sure to note it. Direct quotes help.

Stressful Circumstances

Jail is stressful. Being pulled away from normal events is stressful. Coming into jail the first time is stressful. But coming into jail the fourth or fifth time is not nearly so stressful. Inmates may be unhappy at the interruption of their lives, but by now they know the drill. The jail is a familiar place for them. If they are acting as if they are having a major meltdown over the fact of being incarcerated and they have been in jail over and over, it may all simply be an act, a way of trying to pry drugs out of you. Many inmates are unhappy to learn that benzodiaze-pines, doxepin, hydroxyzine, diphenhydramine, mirtazapine, quetiapine, and trazodone are not available to them.

Prenatal Influences

We will begin our diagnoses by starting at the beginning. Many inmates have issues that stem from before and during childhood; ignoring those issues nets you an incorrect diagnosis. The more studies that are done, the more early childhood looms as not simply a stressor, but a determinant of diagnosis. This is actually part of our cultural heritage: the saying "As a twig is bent so grows the tree" comes from somewhere.

Getting a history of maternal drug or alcohol use allows you to conclude with varying degrees of certainty that an inmate suffered from F88 (315.8) {6A0Y} Neurodevelopmental Disorder—Prenatal Alcohol Exposure (ND-PAE; DSM-5 appendix) to Fetal Alcohol Spectrum Disorder Q86 FASD (760.71) {KA06.2, LD2F.00}; but the latter codes have more to do with dysmorphic features than they do with behavioral disturbances. F88 (315.8) {6A0Y} covers Other Disorders of Psychological Development but it includes ND-PAE. A recent study published in JAMA found fetal alcohol spectrum disorders (including ND-PAE) in 222 of 6639 children, representing a rate of 11-50 cases per 1000 births in the US. At least one commenter cites evidence that this is a gross underestimate.

According to current research, women using cocaine also abuse alcohol, and this exposure means that a "crack baby" is actually an alcohol-exposed baby—with at least ND-FAE, and maybe even FASD. These people tend to have ADHD symptoms emphasizing irritability, and impulsivit, with other signs of impaired self-regulation and impaired biopsychological development (BIF or ID in some cases). In DSM-IV, the prenatal exposure diagnoses are coded on Axis III. In DSM-5 there are no axes.

Abuse, Early Trauma

Moving on to a history of abuse, we learn what kind of traumas the inmate experienced from early in her life. She will tell you about traumas from earliest childhood to adulthood, but stop her after adolescence. Here we are more concerned with her developmental history. And pay particular attention to who the inmate told about the abuse. Was she too afraid to tell anyone? Did she tell someone who hushed her up? Then make some inquiries into ongoing symptoms, but keep the line of questions limited; we have a lot of ground to cover and we don't need to have an inmate breaking down in mid-interview.

Sometimes, though, you have little choice. Case after case of people show up who have been mightily abused in childhood (e.g.—the woman whose mother rented her out for sex from 3-10 years old) or mightily traumatized in childhood (e.g.—the boy who at 6 years old saw his father shot and killed in front of him). Their under-standable cases of reaction formation were diagnosed at the time as "bipolar disorder" in-stead of responses to trauma; they were treated with antipsychotics instead of psychotherapy. If your psychiatric history had been confined to adulthood, you would have missed the key elements of the case.

When you consider reactions to the kinds of trauma that many inmates were exposed to when they were children (ACE's), the concept of ICD-9

309.81 PTSD hardly covers the situations; ICD-10 F43.12 chronic PTSD might be a better fit. In ICD-11 we finally have a specific code for Complex PTSD {6B41}:

"ICD-11 CPTSD includes the three PTSD clusters and three additional clusters that reflect 'disturbances in self-organization' (DSO): (1) affective dysregulation, (2) negative self-concept, and (3) disturbances in relationships. These disturbances are proposed to be typically associated with sustained, repeated, or multiple forms of traumatic exposure (e.g. genocide campaigns, childhood sexual abuse, child soldiering, severe domestic violence, torture, or slavery), reflecting loss of emotional, psychological, and social resources under conditions of prolonged adversity." (Karatzias et al.) The three elements they identify sure look a lot like what has been called borderline personality disorder. Is it any wonder that BPD has been described as complex PTSD?

For people who did not develop a full PTSD picture, the diagnoses of Dysthymia F34.1 (300.4) {6A72} along with BPD F60.3 (301.83) {6D11.5} may be an appropriate collection of diagnoses. When none of these quite fit, F43.2 (309.9) {6B43} Adjustment Disorder NOS (with an explanation in parentheses) will have to do. But you will note that in ICD-10, we still do not have a direct diagnosis for someone's responses to ACE's. ICD-11 finally addresses this lack.

ADHD and Special Ed

After getting the abuse history, you will find yourself in the inmate's adolescence. Time to circle back and ask about ADHD symptoms and special education. In earlier times, special education was reserved for "slow learners" (i.e.—cognitively limited students) but for the past two or three decades, depending on the school district, special education has been used for children who have special learning needs, and for those with disruptive behavior. For our purposes, a history of special ed is a flag. When the inmate says he was in special ed, had special classes, a child study team (CST) or was in a resource room, it is often a signal that says the school noticed his ADHD. So, ask questions about the inmate's taking Ritalin, Concerta, Adderall or Vyvanse (all trademarked) when he was young. These can lead to a diagnosis of F90 (314.01) {6A05} ADHD. Also expect inmates who have ADHD to complain of lying awake at night and sleeping late into the morning, unable to get up for morning meds. These complaints are normal for ADHD, and are not symptoms of depression.

Mood Instability—DMDD

DSM-5 added a valuable diagnosis to the armamentarium of psychiatrists who treat children—F34.81 (296.99) {6C90.0Z} Disruptive Mood Dysregulation Disorder (DMDD). The "core feature" is "chronic, severe persistent irritability." Patients have frequent temper tantrums. You will have histories of many an inmate who was diagnosed "bipolar" and treated with often-heroic doses of antipsychotic drugs in childhood. ICD-11 categorizes these children as having "Oppositional defiant disorder with chronic irritability-anger, unspecified" {6C90.0Z}; call it DMDD.

Seen from afar, these children look like they have ADHD and IED, not bipolar disorder. DMDD is actually distinct from bipolar disorder, IED and ADHD. If you look at the subsequent history, some children will have both ADHD and DMDD but not bipolar disorder. Bipolar disorder almost always begins in adolescence, so when an inmate has mood instability or anger outbursts (recurrent tantrums) starting in childhood, they most likely have something other than bipolar disorder. Having the new diagnosis of DMDD allows for more diagnostic clarity and perhaps better treatment for your inmates. Consider also ND-PAE and cPTSD here.

Many inmates who have a history of DMDD also have a history of ADHD, and a history of abuse or other trauma in childhood. Not only have they had houses burn down, they have witnessed their mothers being beaten; they have suffered as parents, stepparents or foster parents put them down verbally or were purposely cruel to them. Children labeled with DMDD or ODD or IED or BD might have been responding to hurts at home (ACE's), but the clinicians treating them never asked, and no one told those clinicians.

See also pp 99-100 for more on DMDD.

Intellectual Disability and Borderline Intellectual Functioning

If your inmate seems to have less intellectual capacity than normal, do ask *Did kids tease you for being slow? Can you read and write?* And *Are you on Disability?* The answers to these questions can lead to a diagnosis of F70 (317) {6A00.Z} Intellectual Disability (ID) or R41.83 (V62.89) Borderline Intellectual Functioning (BIF) (ICD-11 intends to lump this one in with ID; we'll see). Making these diagnoses is important because they speak to an inmate's 'cognitive reserve,' his intellectual capacity for learning to cope with stress.

Let's be clear here: intellectual disability is not a mental illness; it simply describes a dimension of a person, like weight. Healthcare workers must adjust their treatment to whether a person has normal weight or is obese. Similarly, mental healthcare workers adapt their care to whether a person has normal intellectual capacity or is intellectually disabled. But intellectual disability is not an 'illness' that can be treated—meds cannot make someone smart. And note that ICD-9 listed BIF as a V code (factors that influence health status or describe contact with health services, describing reasons for encounter other than for disease or injury). ICD-10 lists BIF in a section that "excludes symptoms and signs constituting part of a pattern of mental disorder." Below-normal intellectual functioning is clearly not a mental illness *per se,* though it can affect mental illness through its crippling of cognitive reserve.

Substances

Since a lot of inmates start their substance abuse with adolescence, now is a reasonable time to ask for this history. Usually a colleague will ask about these, so you can glance at the substance abuse history in the Mental Health Intake or whatever it is called at your jail. But the important elements—and you may have to ask about these yourself—are *when* the inmate began abusing substances and whether they were downers or uppers. For diagnostic purposes, an inmate can have one or two substance dependence issues (e.g.—Alcohol Dependence F10.2 (303.9) {6C40.2} and Cannabis Dependence F12.2 (304.3) {6C41.2}) but if they have been dependent on three or more substances, in ICD-9 you can diagnose 304.8 Polysubstance Dependence and move on. In DSM-5 there is no concept of dependence, which is sad. In ICD-10 the substance code F1x.2 specifies substance dependence; but there is no analogous code for multiple substances. I recommend you use F19.2 Other psychoactive substance dependence and note it as Polysubstance Dependence (PSD). In ICD-11, I recommend {6C4F.2} Multiple specified psychoactive substances dependence.

As I noted before, you normally won't have time to dwell on details; but occasionally you will have some spare moments to listen to details. So, for example, one can learn that an inmate with ADHD experiences a calming effect with methamphetamine or cocaine at moderate doses; or that he felt stimulated when he used opiates (both characteristic of ADHD).

A person develops substance dependence when he cannot function without it. When an addict feels anything—happy, sad, scared, mad— he reaches for the bottle, the blunt or the needle. DSM-5 has abandoned the concept of dependence and instead calibrates various levels of abuse. This was an unfortunate editorial decision on their part, because it leaves clinicians without a means of denoting a person who is likely to relapse and has psychodynamic "needs"—like using substances as a defense against normal stressors. The only justification is to note that the DSM is a Diagnostic and Statistical Manual; the statistics of abuse are easier to tabulate than concepts of dependence.

Also consider whether the inmate is withdrawing or detoxing from substances. You can note these conditions in your impression, or put it under Axis III if you are still using DSM-IV. The importance of Detox of course is that the inmate may be having "anxiety" and "depression" from something that is not a mental illness but from her withdrawing or detoxing from drugs. It is our job to help with the former (mental illnesses) and let the medical department help her with the latter (withdrawal and detox).

Medical Issues

As you might anticipate this is a complex set of issues. But as physicians we have to do an independent inquiry, in case the physical medical providers missed something or the inmate failed to tell the medical providers something. You may also wish to inquire into issues that are beyond what a GP will ask about. Finally, you need to show to the inmate that you are taking his medical condition into account when you treat him.

TBI Recall that we ask about MVA's and TBI's. A special niche is reserved for head injuries and seizures. If an inmate relates a history of a head injury or a concussion, it is prudent to ask if the person was unconscious (LOC) and for how long. If the inmate has a seizure problem, does she have epilepsy, an enduring seizure disorder from childhood? Or perhaps seizures due to head injuries? Perhaps he had a worsening of memory or the onset of ADHD symptoms then.

Seizures and Seizure-Like Activity One interesting aspect of cerebral pathology is the diverse etiology from prenatal exposure to drugs and/or alcohol (F88/315.8 ND-PAE) to TBI's (traumatic brain injuries) suffered in childhood, to seizure disorders of diverse etiology to TBI's suffered in adulthood. In these circumstances, look for behavioral dysregulation, hyperactivity, impulsivity, impulsive violence and gaps in memory. Also, such people may have a pathology associated with the temporal lobes—Temporal-Limbic Dysfunction (TLD), also called Interictal Personality Disorder and Geschwind Syndrome. One may have a temporal aura or the interictal personality often seen in TLE. You can ask the inmate if he smells out-of-place smells (like something sweet or something burning when everyone should smell like body odor) or frequent episodes of deja vu (*Do you have a little deja vu, a lot of deja vu or no deja vu?*). Sometimes patients hear music. Rarely do you see full-blown TLE or partial complex seizures.

Having inmates "black out" when they get angry—lose memory when they have an episode of violence—is unverifiable; you only have an inmate's word for it. After quizzing a large number of inmates about their blackout rages I came to the conclusion that getting a history of post-rage somnolence took too much time and the results were not reliable. Further, the inform-ation lacked validity—it had no predictive value. So, a post-hoc attempt to find out if episodes of violence were partial complex seizures or psych-omotor seizures is fruitless at this time.

Diabetes Don't let diabetes slip by you. This is one of the terrible potential consequences of using second-generation antipsychotic medications. Also, diabetes renders one more likely to develop dementia.

Obesity Do comment on this, on what you see. Ask about it:

When did you gain weight?

You are fishing for weight gain from child-hood, which may be a flag for early history of abuse (abused girls will make themselves obese, hoping their unattractiveness will discourage their abusers); or weight gain during adulthood from such causes as overeating or pregnancy; or weight gain as a consequence of taking second generation antipsychotics.

Tremors may be characterized as resting tremors or action tremors. The assessment of tremors is beyond the scope of this book but you should look again at this subject. A coarse resting tremor that is extinguished on action is often a Parkinsonian or pseudo-parkinsonian tremor. The latter is of course an EPS side effect. A tremor that is greater on extension is more likely to be an essential tremor, a withdrawal tremor or a tremor from lithium treatment.

Only a minority of tremors are psychogenic; but tremors due to anxiety are the first thing an inmate thinks about when he observes a tremor. When you get the complaint of tremor or shakes, unpack the inmate's usage, diagnose the tremor appropriately, refer the inmate appropriately or (in the case of EPS side effects) treat the tremor as a side effect. Only occasionally will you need to treat the tremor as part of a psychiatric illness.

Sleep Apnea (OSAS) The cardinal symptoms of sleep apnea are loud snoring and daytime drowsiness. The full condition usually requires a sleep study for diagnosis but there are less expensive substitutes. The main issue for psychiatrists in sleep apnea is that it can cause a depression that is resistant to psychiatric interventions—medications, therapy, ECT. The best treatment for depression caused by sleep apnea is treatment of the sleep apnea.

Recent research has also found that more than half of people with combat-associated PTSD have sleep apnea. This would suggest that for optimal treatment of their PTSD, their sleep apnea should be addressed. A psychiatrist must now wonder how far this finding applies to people who have suffered non-combat PTSD. Certainly the circumstances involving abuse and domestic violence may be similar to those of a combat environment. Here is where you begin to realize that an attention to early history may guide your treatment decisions.

You should always have a high index of suspicion for sleep apnea. As an example, I recently interviewed an inmate who wanted to restart paroxetine for panic attacks. He snored at night and during the daytime he was tired, sleepy. This had come on him in the last decade or two. He ate a lot of sugar to keep himself awake. The panic attacks had started about 15 years ago. He used to go to ER's because he thought he was having heart attacks. He did not like most meds for panic attacks because they made him drowsy—even SSRI's. An observer noted he stopped breathing at times during sleep. After I made the suggestion of OSAS-related SOB which would wake him from sleep, he noted that he had GERD and slept upright. This also reduced his "panic attacks." He was able to connect various problems once the diagnosis was proposed to him. He noted, for example, that he was awakened from sleep with these panic attacks; they generally did not bother him during the day. So we turned a psychiatric issue into a medical issue. He would get a sleep study as soon as he left jail. In the meantime I restarted his paroxetine. Hopefully, this clinical example will reinforce the need for getting a medical history.

HPI (History of the Present Illness; Psychiatric History)

The reason for establishing the immediacy of an inmate's suicidal behavior and history of psychiatric admissions is to help you render a decision on whether the inmate needs special precautions to be taken or immediate medication or both. Also if you have a middle-class inmate who developed his psychiatric illness in adolescence or adulthood this is where the psychopathology is centered. To address specific syndromes:

Anxiety

(See also Appendix G.)

Inmates may say they are "anxious." Those who have never been to jail before can be fearful—they may worry about what is going to happen to them. Inmates who have been to jail before but worry about things going on outside the jail may say they are "anxious." They may be fearful. They may worry. But they do not have anxiety. They are having understandable, even appropriate responses to incarceration. Normal responses to adverse circumstances do not add up to a mental illness. Instead they are Z65.1 (V62.5) {QE41} a normal response to jail.

Inmates often say they have "anxiety" when they have symptoms of ADHD. They complain that they "can't sit still," they have "racing thoughts" and "can't focus." Sometimes they have symptoms of essential tremor and from that they conclude that they must be anxious. In the middle of withdrawal from alcohol or drugs they have the shakes and feel bad; they say they feel "anxious." None of these people have anxiety *per se*. They may have ADHD, essential tremor or withdrawal symptoms. They may even feel anxious at the moment. But they do not have the mental disorder called 'anxiety.'

Anxiety and fear are related, but new research shows that they light up different portions of the brain. Fear is the emotional response that people have to dangerous things. Fear of perceived danger is not anxiety, it is fear. Fear of danger or fear of potentially dangerous situations is a response that helped our ancestors survive dangerous situations. Ignoring fear can kill you. But anxious people have undirected anticipation of danger. They are excessively alert, apprehensive of what, they do not know—in essence, scared in all directions. This is dysfunctional, because while they are busy being afraid of everything, they can miss real danger from a particular something. So anxiety disorders deserve to be treated by outside doctors, both psychologists and psychiatrists. It is less clear that anxiety should be treated by jail psychiatrists.

People with ADHD are more likely than others to develop real anxiety, so you may encounter inmates who "treat" this with drugs—which worsen their anxiety with time. Of course this is ironic, but anxious drug addicts are strongly motivated to return to their drugs, using their anxiety as an excuse to continue their addictions. Marijuana users figure prominently in this.

If the anxiety is among the symptoms of an ongoing depression, then that symptom will be treated when you treat the depression. But the inmate could have been taking a benzodiazepine or quetiapine as an adjunct, or even as the primary treatment for a depression. In that case one treats the inmate as if she is withdrawing from a drug, since she is.

Some inmates will tell you they often have a heavy chest. This may be a symptom of anxiety. Some complain of feeling "nervous" with sweaty palms when they are around people. This of course is social phobia, but it can be part of a

PTSD cluster, so a careful history is important. More on both later.

Sometimes an inmate presents as having an anxiety disorder that was treated before she came to jail. You take a history and conclude that the symptoms are consistent with anxiety. But you know that inmates lie and this inmate—like many inmates—may be stringing you along, lying to you. You don't know if she really has anxiety or not. What to do? You write down the diagnosis. If you can, you get reports from staff who have observed the inmate when she did not know she was under observation, or observed her when she did not expect that the CO she was talking to would ever report the observations to you. But even if you can't get that information, you treat the inmate in ways that make her lying to you a fruitless endeavor. You will prescribe no comfort pills. You will refer her for group or individual psychotherapy if that is available. Among chemicals, you will treat her only with SSRI's, buspirone, duloxetine or venlafaxine—no diphenhydramine, doxepin, hydroxyzine, mirtaza-pine or trazodone. With no drugs forthcoming, only medications, the inmate will either stick with the psychological treatment and/or take the prescribed medications; or the inmate will drop off your census, disappointed.

Depression

Many inmates complain of depression, and come to the psychiatrist asking for a chemical to help with their feeling down. It may not be clear if an inmate is suffering from a depressive illness or simply unhappy with his or her circumstances, but inmates still come looking for chemical help. Of course, most don't care if you give them a drug or a medicine. Any chemical will do. It might as well be magic—but that is for another discussion.

The most common psychiatric diagnoses are depression and anxiety. Lucky for us that the treatment for both lies in the same class of medications: the SSRI's. As added bonuses, SSRI's cannot be abused and are not fatal in overdose. This was not the case for the prior generation of antidepressants, the TCA's. While those were effective in about 80% of patients with "endogenous" or major depression, they were less effective with dysthymia. Worse, they caused weight gain and cardiac abnormalities; when they were used properly, TCA's were the leading cause of death by overdose. Yes, it is ironic but true.

Even today, an outpatient psychiatric provider might spend a lot of time distinguishing between a major depression and a dysthymia. A lot of this is due to reimbursement issues, freedom from which is an advantage for jail shrinks. But a major issue is this: you don't harm inmates by treating their unhappiness with an SSRI, whether they technically have a depression or not. Further, an inmate who is not suffering from the number of symptoms required to formally diagnose depression may still be suffering. It would be cruel to withhold an SSRI under such circumstances.

Perhaps the sole reason for totting up depressive symptoms is so you can keep track of how the patients are progressing. Sometimes they say they're worse; but compared with your record of how they were doing, they may have improved. Of course, they are better liars than you are a lie detector. While you were learning to doctor to patients, they were learning to lie to everyone. So you can't really trust what an inmate tells you.

When I have run psych units, I have quietly observed patients; and staff reported to me how particular patients were doing, so I could have a good feel for how a patient was functioning. But in a jail, you have the reports of CO's, who medically are lay people. And worse: often you cannot get even a layperson's report on how she is doing from a CO that knows the inmate, be-cause the jail is always shifting personnel.

One way of distinguishing major depression from an adjustment disorder or grief is to observe whether the inmate can smile and laugh spontaneously and appropriately. It has long been known that distracting someone from his grief can allow you to make him laugh. This is one reason I insert into my inquiry "Who do you want to kill?" and other bald questions. They can start-le inmates out of their depressive stance and allow their underlying mental state to shine through. A truly depressed person can't laugh.

Bottom line: if an inmate complains of de-pression, you will usually treat her with an antidepressant. If it doesn't work, she will ask for a different med. If an inmate is looking for a drug, the fact that she can only get medicines discourages her; she quits taking all meds and drops off your census. Because it doesn't matter what kind of a depression an inmate has, it shortens the inquiry and simplifies your diagnosis. The common diagnosis is F32.9 (311) {6A7Z} Depression NOS, which is the code you use when you cannot obtain enough reliable information to make a diagnosis beyond the fact that the inmate has some kind of depression. You may wish to document some uncertainty. You can do that: F32.9 Depression NOS (put your uncertainty within parentheses).

Other depressive disorders include: F43.21 (309.0) {6B42} Adjustment Disorder with Depressed Mood—note that 43.2 is the only F43 code that does *not* refer to a "severe stress." F43.2 (309.9) {6B43} Adjustment Disorder NOS refers to an excessive response to a normal life stressor. It may be better to use Z65.1 {QE41} here (Normal Reaction to Incarceration): incarceration is a large stressor, and not a normal life event. Pathological grief is an example of adjustment disorder with depressed mood in ICD-10, coded as F43.21.

Another depressive disorder is F34.1 (300.4) {6A72} Dysthymia (Neurotic Depression or Depressive Neurosis). But do not use F32 (296.2) {6A70.3 and sequellae} Major Depression or F33 (296.3) {6A71.1} Recurrent Major Depression— you won't have enough reliable history to diagnose those.

Remember that opiate use by itself can cause depression, as can alcohol use; so can cocaine withdrawal. For substance users who are depressed, you have no way of knowing whether the inmate was using opiates because he was depressed or depressed because he was using opiates. If you just treat the depression with an SSRI, it won't matter.

Oh yes: if an inmate complains of not sleeping, look at him. Does he seem that short of sleep? Sleepless people have a certain haggard look. A person with ADHD may complain of initial insomnia, lying awake at night with "racing thoughts," a concept that was taught to the public by well-meaning psychiatrists. This is not a symptom of depression; people with depression wake in the middle of the night. People with initial insomnia do not usually suffer from lack of sleep; they tend to stay up late and sleep late, missing morning med time. Instead, learning the rudiments of sleep hygiene will help them learn to get up in the morning and stay awake all day so they will feel like going to sleep at night. There is no need for psychiatric intervention in these cases.

One last thing on sleep: if you go to the trouble of having people observe inmates who complain they "can't sleep" they often see them snoring away. Another thing you can do is examine sleep logs. Almost all inmates are fast asleep.

Be wary when you come across someone with TRD (treatment-resistant depression). The inmate may have dysthymia. One thing will strike you as you read papers on TRD across the decades: the observation that a third of de-pressed patients do not respond to any therapy seems modeled on middle class people, and not people who have undergone chronic trauma like concentration camp survivors or people who were abused as children. When you have a patient who seems to have TRD, you should look at her early history. You might find something treatable there, but usually not with meds.

Dysthymia

Dysthymia is usually a lifelong disorder, with its onset in childhood. Often you will find that the inmates have suffered beatings and molestations. They have been called liars or beaten by their caregivers for reporting the abuse, whether to their mothers or to authorities. Sometimes this condition is mistaken for persistent depression, leading to treatment with meds, or even ECT.

Emotional dysregulation and unstable moods are a hallmark of 'neurotic depression' or F34.1 (300.4) {6A72} Dysthymia. Good days, bad days, emotional ups and downs, angry feelings, anxieties—these are all typical of dysthymia. People with this condition typically over-respond to circumstances whether happy or unhappy, but especially unhappy. Although they do respond to SSRI's, they do best with psychotherapy. For people with borderline personality disorder: if DBT is available, that is a good option for them.

They may have "bipolar" disorder but they certainly do not have bipolar disorder.

Another issue is the confusion of dysthymia and DSM-5 Persistent Depression. They are not the same thing. A persistent depression can arise in adolescence or adulthood and is frustratingly hard to treat. A dysthymia usually arises in childhood from a difficult or even abusive experience. People with dysthymia have an unstable mood. People with persistent depression have a stable but low mood.

"Bipolar Disorder"

The example neatly leads to a discussion of "bipolar disorder" and bipolar disorder. Bipolar disorder is a real psychiatric disorder. It has been known from early times. The term 'lunatic' refers to the belief that sufferers became "crazy" during certain phases of the moon. If you have ever taken care of real bipolars on inpatient units or in outpatient practices, you know they can be difficult to treat. A bipolar in his depressed phase can be difficult to treat because some of our most effective antidepressants can and do destabilize bipolar patients, provoking manic or mixed episodes. Lucky for us, the incidence of bipolar disorder is only 2-3% of the general population.

Of course, these days "bipolar disorder"—as opposed to bipolar disorder—is an epidemic. Because there remain few antidepressants on patent, drug companies no longer push the diagnosis of depression. Instead, they push "bipolar disorder" and some of the most expensive medications on the market—second-generation antipsychotics. These medications also can cause diabetes, weight gain, dyslipidemia and hyper-prolactinemia separately and simultaneously. It is no wonder that the metabolic syndrome is suddenly a concern for us: our new antipsychotic medicines *cause* the metabolic syndrome.

A more insidious motivator is managed care. If your managed care patient merely has a depression, you file a treatment plan and the care manager wants to know when you will cure the person and get her off your caseload. Bipolar disorder, on the other hand, is known to be genetic; it is a biological disorder that never quits. So the patient is called "bipolar disorder" and the doctor is left alone. The unfortunate patient is in for a life of treatment, and the care manager cannot object. Similarly, for a rehab program finding a case of "bipolar disorder" makes the billing more certain. Not that I would suggest that these programs deliberately misdiagnose their patients (heaven forfend) but the temptation is definitely there.

This is not to say that all detox programs operate this way. Some programs are staffed with well-meaning psychiatrists who see that patients appear active on SSRI's so they diagnose "bipolar disorder." What those doctors are forgetting is that they are treating people in the withdrawal and detox phases of coming off drugs. You can't get a good diagnosis when body or brain is screaming for its missing substance. Even during the rehab phase following detox, an inmate can show "mood swings" (they are actually fluctuations in mood) that can be damped with divalproex. Diagnosis of "bipolar" in such circumstances is fraught with error. A good rule of thumb is to withhold the diagnosis for a year after an inmate has quit substances. Otherwise the process moves from diagnosis to overdiagnosis.

The overdiagnosis has gotten so pervasive and so bad that lay people now think that "bipolar disorder" means unstable mood. They think they need quetiapine and clonazepam—both drugs of abuse, even though they are both legal (notice I used 'and' there). When SSRI's are prescribed, they believe those meds are "mood stabilizers," not antidepressants.

Sometimes people with emotional dysregulation are called "bipolar 2." For the record, the concept of F31.81 (296.89) {6A61.Z} Bipolar II Disorder was created when psychiatrists were treating cases of depression with tricyclic antidepressants and were surprised when their depressed patients suddenly became manic or hypomanic. This uncovering of bipolar disorder by an antidepressant was the hallmark of the bipolar II disorder. The term should not cover people who merely have emotional dysregulation and unstable moods.

One way to determine whether an inmate has bipolar disorder or bipolar 2 is to treat his depression with an antidepressant. Another is stress: stress often produces manic episodes.

Antidepressants—if unopposed by 'mood stabilizers' like divalproex—can produce manic or mixed episodes, especially SNRI's like venlafaxine and duloxetine, and TCA's like amitriptyline. If the inmate is in jail for months, under enormous stress and taking an antidepressant, you would expect her to crack up and become manic—if she indeed has a bipolar disorder. In the event, very few inmates crack because they do not truly have bipolar disorders. They have "bipolar disorder" which can be an episode of depression, part of a dysthymia, an adjustment disorder, borderline personality disorder or simply a normal reaction to an unhappy circumstance; and incarceration is just such an unhappy circumstance.

Emotional dysregulation and unstable moods are typical in cases of dysthymia—'neurotic depression' as it was called before DSM-III. An even earlier term was 'depressive neurosis.' Even when people have major depression, they have good days and bad days. Good days, bad days, emotional ups and downs, angry feelings, anxieties; these are all typical of dysthymia and have nothing to do with the hypomanic, manic or mixed episodes seen in true bipolar disorder. And don't forget the mood dysregulation seen in complex PTSD.

F34.81 (296.99) {6C90.0Z} Disruptive Mood Dysregulation Disorder (**DMDD**) is characterized by persistent irritability—severe irritability with frequent tantrums. Children can act out verbally and physically. The types of negative feedback given to such children in the past are now frowned upon, so such children have few firm limits to run up against; their behavior goes wild. Before DSM-5, clinicians would often give such wild children the diagnosis of "bipolar" and dope them up. Sometimes a child who has had serious traumatic experiences and acts out is also given the diagnosis of "bipolar." No one asks the kid about trauma.

But incarceration can happen to anyone. You don't have to be mentally ill to get put in jail (though some would argue that it helps). If someone is unhappy to suddenly find herself in jail, complaining of "mood swings" and "bipolar disorder" she does not have bipolar disorder. Yes, she is upset. But she is having a normal response to an upsetting event—Z65.1 (V62.5) {QE41} incarceration, imprisonment.

Consider age of onset. People with the unstable mood disorder usually complain of unstable moods and sensitivity to events going back to childhood. Actual bipolar disorder almost always has its onset in late adolescence or early adulthood. So when you find an inmate telling you he has "bipolar disorder" going back to childhood you can diagnose F43.12 (309.81) Chronic PTSD, {6B41} Complex PTSD, F34.81 (296.99) {6C90.0Z} DMDD, F34.1 (300.4) {6A72} dysthymia, or all three.

Finally, consider: many of your patients come to you taking divalproex and an antipsychotic. They are dulled but they are still depressed. Their "bipolar disorder" is being treated but not their depression. You can do a real service by switching them to an SSRI.

Bipolar Disorder

On the other hand an inmate who is active and hostile, with a blunted affect and an expansive demeanor; who has loud pressured speech with odd grandiose ideas; is either intoxicated or manic. He may have bipolar disorder—the real thing. Unfortunately, the police are bringing mentally ill people to jail, and a number of jails lack the ability to turn away police who are bringing mentally ill people to their doors. So the jail's mental health team will have to deal with them. The codes for bipolar disorder episodes range widely, as you can infer from the wide spread of bipolar codes in ICD-9 (look them up if you don't believe me); the ICD-10 diagnostic scheme for bipolar disorder is much more complicated than the diagnostic scheme for DSM-IV/ICD-9. Here is where you can clearly see that ICD is a billing codeset, not aimed at clinicians. The jail shrink's response is to diagnose F31 {6A6Z} and keep going.

To diagnose bipolar disorder, listen for the psychiatric admissions where the inmate was hospitalized against his will for reasons he does not understand, reasons that do not make sense, or explanations involving other people being unhappy with his behavior. Remember that when a person is manic he often will have gaps in his memory for manic symptoms. If someone has not been hospitalized with a manic episode, a diagnosis of "bipolar disorder" should be greeted with deep skepticism. But if a patient's list of symptoms sounds like she has been having manic episodes, make sure they last four days before you decide the inmate actually has bipolar disorder.

Doctors often use excess shopping as their proxy for manic episodes. They consider shopping sprees to be pathognomonic manic behavior. Unfortunately, shopping sprees are often used by neurotic people as a defense against unhappiness. Shopping is like a drug for them. So you have to ask about the judgment that accompanied the shopping sprees of the people you are talking to (even for neurotics, their mood will be up; their affect and energy will be high).

There is some controversy over whether unexpected surges of energy represent manic episodes or something else. Given that these "surges" last minutes, at most, they probably represent something neurotic, not psychotic. These micro-episodes may simply be the fluctuations of dysthymia. Your colleagues may be in a rush to diagnose "bipolar disorder" here, but that is likely shortchanging the inmate you are talking to. The inmate may cling to the diagnosis of "bipolar," but you should not.

Bipolar disorder usually has its onset in late adolescence. While a lifetime of unstable mood does not prevent someone from developing bipolar disorder, a dysregulated mood state that is essentially unchanged from a disturbed child-hood is not a true bipolar disorder.

Schizophrenia

Although schizophrenia is often thought to be the classic diagnosis of psychiatry, this chronic illness was not known in antiquity. There are indications from national hospital records that it slowly invaded England (and then Europe and the US) from around 1500, reaching its current level after 1900 (see *The Invisible Plague* by Fuller Torrey). Be that as it may, the state hospital systems grew in this country, coming to serve about 1-2% of the population in the years prior to the advent of antipsychotic meds. After that, the hospitals emptied their patients out into the streets, closing their doors behind them, and eventually closing the hospitals themselves, so that there were no longer asylums to shelter the chronic mentally ill. These days, when schizo-phrenics break the law, they are taken not to hospitals but to jails where jailhouse shrinks must take care of them. That means you.

The most severe and chronic cases of schizo-phrenia seem to begin with signs showing up in childhood. This is why when you are dealing with someone who has a blunted affect you add to your history a question on whether the inmate was a loner or socialized with friends during childhood. You can also ask—if the inmate is male—whether the inmate had girlfriends in high school. As the affected inmate ages, his or her psychosis becomes manifest either as a chronic progression, a sudden process, or episodes of psychosis. Remember when you diagnose this, that Bleuler, the man who named this illness 'schizophrenia,' included *autism* in his 'Four A's.' By 'autism' he meant self-involvement, withdrawal into a fantasy world, inability to relate to others, etc.

To get a real feel for the illness, look up and read "The Early Symptoms of Schizophrenia" by James Chapman, British Journal of Psychiatry 112: 225-251 (1966). In addition, look at the inmate's memory. It appears that a person with schizophrenia can relate his history fairly accurately until he became ill. After that, events are often jumbled and conflated. The accuracy of dates and other issues is highly suspect for events that occurred after the inmate became psychotic. For events following the onset of illness, your HPI is likely to be inaccurate. Focusing on the experience of symptoms will be more helpful than focusing on the sequence of events.

Even though there is some suggestion that schizophrenia is actually a collection of perhaps eight conditions, the field is not ready to diagnose them as separate illnesses. The older DSM-IV diagnostic scheme ranges from F20.0 (295.3) Paranoid Schizophrenia—a psychotic process in a patient without a formal thought disorder—to F20.1 (295.1) Disorganized Schizophrenia, also called hebephrenia, which is dominated by cognitive disorganization. In addition, ICD-10 includes F20.6 Simple Schizophrenia and F20.4 Post-Schizophrenic Depression.

DSM-5 rejects the various types because a clinical picture can change over time; in essence, it argues that the types describe not separate disorders reliably ascertained and validly followed, but various phases of a single illness. It simply lists Schizophrenia as an undifferentiated whole. This is F20 in ICD-10 and 295 in ICD-9. The jail shrink would do well to follow DSM-5 here, diagnose F20 (295) {6A2Z} schizophrenia and move on.

Schizophrenic-Seeming Psychoses

A broad or normally responsive affect should put questions in your mind. Such inmates most likely do not have a schizophrenia-related diagnosis. The ability to relate in a personal and emotional way is generally not consistent with a diagnosis of schizophrenia. In particular this is not consistent with *autism*, one of Bleuler's "Four A's" of schizophrenia.

Just because someone has hallucinations and delusions does not make her schizophrenic. A person who has mania may have hallucinations and delusions. So may someone who is intoxicated with a psychotomimetic drug (PCP, for example, can linger in one's adipose tissue). You really make your diagnosis over time. (In fact, there is still some controversy in the field over whether alcohol and drugs can cause psychosis or simply bring out a latent schizophrenia. This debate was ongoing in the 1970's and I don't expect it to get settled soon.) But what should you do? You don't have time to delve deeply into the history of every inmate you see—so diagnose F29 (298.9) {6A2Y} Psychosis NOS—and move on.

There does not appear to be a code for when you see a psychosis but do not know its etiology, mental illness vs toxicity. ICD-10 F09 is for Un-specified Mental Disorder Due To Known Physio-logical Condition and includes an old diagnosis, Organic Brain Syndrome (OBS). It may also apply to toxicosis (e.g.—a poison, or a drug, or thyro-toxicosis). Alas; we are still at sea when we do not know where the psychosis comes from. R69 (799.9) {MG48} Deferred (put your differential in parentheses) may be your best choice.

There are the intrusive thoughts of PTSD. Persons with PTSD may experience intrapsychic voices, hallucinated voices and visions of people and situations they have encountered in the past. These experiences are PTSD-related, and not due to schizophrenia. Again, a normal affect tends to argue against the diagnosis of schizophrenia, although persons with schizophrenia may develop PTSD.

Attention: the distinction is important. With PTSD-related voices you may medicate the psych-osis and not touch the PTSD. Worse, you may erroneously medicate the inmate for psychosis, exposing him to all the potential risks of antipsychotic meds, and never touch his voices, which after all are PTSD-related and not part of a psychosis.

On the other hand, there is some evidence that some real psychoses have their beginning with traumatic episodes. Some schizophrenia, for example, seems to begin with trauma or with TBI. Because these cases do exist, your observations on an inmate's affect will be tremendously valuable.

When you have an inmate who relates with you too well to have schizophrenia, you will want to consider alternatives. For example the inmate may have **PTSD**. But she may also have **TLD**. The more extreme case may qualify as having Geschwind Syndrome or Interictal Personality Disorder, but our inmates may complain of a collection of symptoms from childhood, including their hearing voices, hearing music, holding conversations with objects and unseen others (who may have a name), smelling out-of-place smells, experiencing déjà vu frequently and having emotional lability. Clinically, they may appear to have a combination of ADHD, dysthymia and BPD; yet they have a history of voices if you pry. Often these inmates have taken high potency antipsychotics without silencing their auditory hallucinations. Sometimes something as simple as carbamazepine 200mg BID solves their problems. Diagnostically, this seems to be a puzzle. ICD-10 seems to consider brain problems more severe than this when it enumerates brain and nervous system disorders. F63.9 Unspecified Impulse control Disorder is something that comes close to this diagnosis. Here you can Diagnose F88 (315.8) {6E8Z} and call it Temporal-Limbic Dysfunction (TLD).

Psychosis

Often a formal thought disorder, a disorder in the form or flow of an inmate's thinking, can be a clue that a psychosis is present. However, a seeming flight of ideas (FOI) or a pressure in an inmate's speech may stem from a paranoid psychosis almost as often as from a manic process, so FOI is not a reliable indicator of diagnosis.

Probably the best way to diagnose hallucinations is to start from the definition: a hallucination is a false sensory perception. The inmate cannot tell that he is experiencing a hallucination. To him it sounds, feels and looks like he is experiencing real sensations. Although an experienced schizophrenic might know that he is hearing voices if you ask, the naïve schizophrenic or the psychotic person who does not know he is psychotic will deny that he is hearing voices even as you watch him channeling them. A patient, for example, might hit another person because the patient thinks the other person was saying something, even if someone who was standing next to the patient hears nothing. Also, when you talk to inmates, you occasionally elicit delusions which are told to you as facts—for the inmates these are real experiences.

So don't ask *Do you hear voices?* and *Do you hear things when no one else is present?* Do realize that a truly psychotic person might in all honesty might tell you *No.* Further, you are teaching a malingering inmate what to say. Instead ask *What do people say about you when you walk down the street? What are people saying in a restaurant? What is the TV saying?* This is taking seriously what the inmate is experiencing. Since she acts on her hallucinations, your asking about them is not so very strange.

Psychosis NOS is F29 (298.9) {6A2Y}.

Social Phobia—"Paranoia"

Inmates will tell you they are "paranoid." But when you unpack what they are saying the inmate is describing how when she looks out at a group of people, she is afraid to go out there: the people would disapprove of her. Or another inmate may feel a group of people are talking about him, plotting to do bad things to him; he can't actually hear what they are saying—that would be hallucinating. Note that in both situations the inmate is leery of people they can see, not people they cannot see, unseen powers, nor a government conspiracy. There are no hallucinations involved, simply the idea that the people in the group are an "in crowd" and the inmate is outside it.

This is social phobia, of course. The inmates is not paranoid—a psychotic process—but he fears groups of people, which is a phobic process. F40.1 (300.23) {6B04} Social phobia is so common in the addict population that AA and NA have a process for dealing with it: talking to the group. The fact that attendees are sharing their experiences reinforces the group process. The process of repeatedly talking to a group highlights a technique for dealing with any phobia: systematic desensitization through repetitive confrontation, also called exposure therapy.

PTSD

(See Appendix PT for a fuller discussion.) PTSD is classically represented by a triad of symptom clusters: re-experiencing the traumatic events, avoiding traumatic reminders and a persistent sense of threat, including hypervigilance and excessive startle response.

Post-Traumatic Stress Disorder is a condition that psychiatry is still learning about. It was originally described in the American Civil War. It gained notoriety as "shell shock" in World War I. It was during that conflict that the basic principles involved in treating cases of acute onset PTSD were developed by the French. World War II produced its own cases of PTSD, but they were generally ignored in the population's relief to have the war over. PTSD was ignored after the Korean War as well. Finally, during the Viet Nam War, PTSD became well known to the populace.

Veterans were having dramatic flashbacks, indulging in drugs, drinking excessively, and the VA system was unprepared. Decades later, the VA had lots of new medications to try on the new veterans from the wars in the Middle East. But other than prazosin, which appeared to reduce the intensity of nightmares, no medication actually treated the PTSD. Even prazosin is not wholeheartedly accepted by the VA: they have negative studies on that, too, and cite side effects like hypotension. All psychiatrists could do was to prescribe antidepressants for the concomitant depression, and to prescribe chemicals to calm down a person's moods.

In the decades since Viet Nam, psychiatrists also began to recognize that people could develop PTSD from any of life's stressors. PTSD sufferers were not confined to survivors of the holocaust. People who survived beatings, molestation, criminal attacks, house fires, MVA's—all of these could have F43.1x (309.81) {6B40} PTSD.

PTSD can result in numbing, depression, anxiety and social avoidance, along with re-experiencing trauma and excessive alertness. A rational treatment of depression might be an SSRI like sertraline. A rational treatment of the anxiety might be buspirone. If the inmate is frightened of others (social phobia), you might choose a psychological intervention or venlafaxine.

Your task in a jail setting is *not* to treat PTSD with chemicals. For one thing, some of the inmates coming to you with alleged service-connected PTSD have nothing of the sort. They are drug seeking—Z76.5 (V65.2) {QC30} Malingering, alleging PTSD symptoms so you will prescribe them drugs. They are not interested in mere medications.

As the VA discovered a long time ago, drugs cannot be used to treat PTSD successfully (getting a military history is covered in Appendix MI). (But MDMA is in Phase III trials.)

People who develop PTSD can either be victims or perps. While the latter is not the usual case, it does occur and you should be aware of it. The more usual case involves multiple traumas suffered in childhood and early adolescence. The sufferers develop avoidant behavior, and are easily upset. They are often misdiagnosed as having "bipolar disorder." In fact, they have complex PTSD and need psychotherapy, especially EMDR, which is not as available in jails as it is in the community. But a diagnosis of "bipolar disorder" is a barrier to the sufferer in getting any psychotherapy.

You will see cases of gunshot survivors and victims of other crimes. The victims of domestic violence—often recurrent—are fairly common. Sometimes the long history of domestic violence is layered on top of a history of prolonged abuse in childhood. All of this makes the symptoms of PTSD worse. Inmates may complain of "paranoia," but when you dig a bit, you discover they are afraid that people around them will hurt them. After all, this has been their experience, growing up. In part, this fearfulness is based on past experiences; in part it is based on the fact that the person is surrounded by strangers, criminals. Some of the "paranoia" is reality-based and inmates don't want to be doped up. They want to be able to protect themselves. So don't be in a hurry to call these people psychotic.

PTSD is covered further in Appendix PT.

Borderline Personality Disorder

Back in the early decades of psychoanalysis when some neurotic patients got into therapy, they blew up in apparent psychosis. Such patients were considered to be on the borderline between neurosis and psychosis. After a few decades, the profession came to say that these patients have Borderline Personality Disorder: F60.3 (301.83) {6D11.5}.

Some people consider BPD to be an elaborate form of PTSD, complex PTSD. BPD can also be considered to be a response to adverse circumstances. For example, splitting seems to be the borderline's arranging for her abusers to fight with one another so they will leave her alone. When borderlines have mistrustful relationships with others, it seems to reflect the circumstances of their upbringings.

A borderline usually also has F34.1 (300.4) {6A72} dysthymia, an unstable mood that is excessively sensitive to circumstances, both good and bad. As such, a dysthymia is hardly diagnostic. Someone who has used substances extensively, for example, will show a mood that is excessively sensitive to circumstances. And then there is the condition of dysthymia itself. So, for borderline personality, you must have more than dysthymia alone.

In taking a history, you can look for indicators. For instance, borderlines are famous for cutting and burning themselves, usually recurrently (SIB). Another is their choice of partners. While they are in the throes of their disorder, they often choose abusive partners. Finally, when alone they tend to decompensate, complaining of depression, feeling "scared" and feeling "empty."

Research has shown that borderlines often improve with time, especially in the context of a stable non-abusive relationship. The reason for diagnosing BPD is to steer the person to DBT or other group or individual psychotherapy.

Adjustment Disorders, Grief

When someone has an inordinate response to a normal stressor we call it F43.2x (309.x) {6B43} Adjustment Disorder. However, jail is very stressful, sometimes extremely so. Who could blame someone for getting upset? When someone is responding normally to a stressor, we probably should not diagnose them with an adjustment disorder. Instead a Z code (V code) is more appropriate. You may wish to give your inmate a diagnosis of Z65.1 (V62.5) {QE41} incarceration, imprisonment. Such a diagnosis is not a psychiatric disorder at all, simply a normal response to a stressful situation.

ICD-10 includes grief in Adjustment Dis–order. This is a good thing. But how do you tell the difference between an adjustment disorder and depression? The old guidance was this: when someone is grieving you can break her out of her grief by getting her to forget her loss for a moment. Then she will respond to humor with smiles and laughter. Old time comedians understood this. They would begin their acts with sadness, with the kind of loss a grieving person could relate to. Then they would gradually leaven their acts until the whole audience was laughing, including the grief-stricken. The audience members would literally "forget their sorrows" to laugh with a comedian. In a similar way you can tell who is depressed and who is merely unhappy.

An example: a woman came into her home and found her husband dead on the floor. They had been together 30 years and had several children together. She was distraught and was herself taken to a psychiatric hospital, where she was diagnosed with bipolar disorder and PTSD. Now this is a woman who until this point had never needed nor thought she needed psychiatric care; she was herself an accomplished profession-al. She was given a benzodiazepine and a series of antidepressants, none of which addressed her core sadness. Despite what was arguably some numbing and some intrusive thoughts, she had none of the other symptoms of PTSD to accompany her sadness and sense of loss. She had grief. While she was in the psychiatric hospital, she missed going to court to address some fines so (of course) she was arrested and put in jail. In jail, the psychiatrist validated the seriousness of the trauma of losing a co-parent and losing a longstanding partner in love. Afterward she was able to smile through her tears and left the session happy that she was getting no psychiatric medications. Her diagnosis was grief. In earlier times, the experience of grief would have occasioned counseling by a pastor. It is now relegated to mental health professionals.

OCD

OCD is a disorder and must be distinguished from Obsessive-Compulsive Personality. Actually, in a study of personalities by team of psychologists, Obsessive-Compulsive Personality had a GAF Score close to 100. If you think about it, this makes sense. You want your lawyer, your doctor and your accountant to be diligent, orderly and paying excessive attention to detail. These attributes of the obsessive-compulsive personality make a person into a superior professional. In fact, one of the goals of a good medical school is to inculcate those very values into its future doctors.

People with biological OCD, on the other hand, are often best described as 'weird.' They are not right. Their affect is a bit blunted. Sometimes people with schizophrenia develop OCD.

There are people who have adopted OCD defenses. They usually are suppressing struggles with their past. Obsessive and compulsive symptoms can be seen to be part of their Complex PTSD.

Malingering

Malingering is a species of lying. But you knew that. More particularly, malingering is instrumental behavior. The inmate may be using his allegations of illness or distress as an instrument, as a tool to force the institution to do his bidding. Or she may be crying dreadfully in your office seemingly desperate in her need for some calming influence, a drug, a boon that is within your power as a physician to grant. Heady stuff isn't it? It feeds right into the narcissism which the inmate knows is there. She is counting on it. How disappointed when the inmate learns you have only medicines to prescribe—only meds that take a week or two to work, or more. No drugs, no comfort pills.

If you stop by the women's unit and covertly observe the inmates, you will see this 'distressed' individual functioning well—perfectly comfortable on the pod. Your comfort pills were not needed after all. If you had ordered some hydroxyzine she might have cheeked them and sold them to another inmate.

More troublesome is the inmate who is willing to use his body as an instrument of his will. After all these are people who stick often stick themselves with needles blunted by reuse every day to feed their drug habits. What do they care if they cut themselves? So what if they bleed? If he can just get to the ER, he might be able to score an opiate injection. If he bangs his head on the wall he might—he hopes—get the opportunity to call home, to arrange a hit, or to instruct an accomplice on how to hide evidence. The motivations might be petty, the disturbances can be large.

An inmate may owe people money. In general population, he is pretty sure he will meet his associates, yet he wants to avoid IA (Internal Affairs). He does not want to be known as a snitch. So he agitates, pretends a psychiatric disturbance. He is kept on watch, away from the general population and away from IA.

The first step to uncovering a malingerer is to understand his primary gain and his secondary gain. When you know what he is trying to do consciously and unconsciously you are in a better position to determine whether he has a real psychiatric disorder—and remember that even a malingerer can have a psychiatric disorder. Once you have determined that, you can decide not to engage his malingering as a psychiatric matter and leave his care and treatment to Custody.

For example, many inmates come to the psychiatrist complaining of a "depression." Some are truly depressed. Some are withdrawing from a drug. Some have come to the psychiatrist to get drugs. When the inmate seems to have a case of depression, you can go ahead and treat it with an SSRI. If an inmate hoards the SSRI, she can't overdose with it and do any harm. It also does not give the inmate any satisfaction as a drug. If she detoxes and no longer needs the med she will quit getting up every morning to take it. If she was faking an illness in the hopes of getting a drug she will stop it after a day or two, because it does not conform to her wishes. If she really has a case of depression, she will get up every morning to take this wonderful pill. You have done no harm (the first rule of medical practice) and you have treated illness. It didn't matter to you whether the inmate was malingering or not.

Much is made of malingering. There are daylong courses on the subject. Just remember two things: inmates are better liars than you are a lie detector, and Do No Harm.

It helps if you treat everybody profession–ally. You should do a full diagnosis on every inmate you meet for the first time. If you wish to diagnose malingering, it is coded Z76.5 (V65.2) {QC30}.

Summary

This survey of the most frequently encount-ered conditions a jailhouse shrink will meet is necessarily incomplete. You will find yourself unconsciously adding to the conditions listed here. Develop your diagnostic acumen and your coding skills. And just remember that "chemical imbalance" is a myth used to sell drugs. The brain is far more complicated than that.

Chapter 6
Substance Abuse

Substances and Addiction—an Overview

A 'substance' is short for 'substance of abuse:' any chemical used to change the mental state of the user right now. A person may alter her states as an occasional recreation or as part of a habit. Use of a substance becomes 'abuse' of a substance when that use causes the inmate some problem(s) or causes some problem(s) to the community.

One may argue that using marijuana is harmless (though evidence is accumulating that it is harmful), we will see later that using any drug is not harm-free. But using heroin or cocaine involves the user in murderous conspiracies. Around 85% of the world's heroin comes from areas in Afghanistan that are under control of the Taliban. Some portion of a heroin user's money, then, supports the killing of American and Afghan soldiers as well as Afghan civilians. If someone uses cocaine, his money partly goes to drug cartels in Mexico that are killing Mexican citizens and getting into gunfights with the government.

Note that these murders do not include the killings that may occur in the US as drug gangs battle for turf. Also, the hostile climate in Mexico and Central America produced by these cartels drives some persons to come to this country illegally, taking low-skilled jobs, jobs that would otherwise go to released inmates. So society has a stake in suppressing illegal drug use. Since using and selling drugs brings people to jail, you will be seeing cases of drug use and abuse.

Drinking alcohol is not illegal *per se*. However, intoxication with alcohol can cause trouble or leads people to commit actions that get them in trouble with the police. Then the police bring them to jail.

Clinically, we do not worry so much about recreational substance users. We shall concern ourselves mainly with habitual users of sub–stances. Habitual use of a substance often leads to dependency on that substance. Dependency is a pattern of habitual abuse where the user cannot cope with life unless he uses his substance or substances on a recurrent basis.

Maturity. Narcotics Anonymous focuses on that issue when members say "You stop growing up when you start picking up." When counselors run groups with incarcerated alcoholics and drug addicts, they note that their mostly clean inmates are acting like adolescents—exactly as you would predict if they stopped growing up when they began their substances in early adolescence. As for the mechanism, consider the metaphor of the weight room: if you lift weights you will get stronger. If a machine lifts the weights for you, the weights get lifted, but you do not get stronger.

This, then, is the core reason that recurrent use of a substance is bad for people: they forgo the daily challenges that build character. Even marijuana can calm a person down. After a tough day interacting with angry customers, a young man can come home and smoke half a joint to calm down. Has he learned to deal with angry customers? No. And when he gets older, he will not know how to deal with angry customers, avoiding them by blowing them all away in a cloud of smoke—until he needs to cope with situations and can no longer avoid them. Then he will get "depressed" and he will be diagnosed "bipolar" and at some point he may come to see you in jail. With our population, the usual amount is a blunt—a cigar shell stuffed with cannabis— or more. The problems then are that much worse.

Disease or automatic behavior? The 12-step programs call addiction a disease. But what develops in the substance-dependent person is worse than a disease: it is automatic behavior. It is a learned response, a complex conditioned reflex that is like riding a bicycle; once you have learned to do it you never forget how. Because acquiring and using a substance is a complex conditioned reflex, it represents motor learning; and the behavior can be exercised without the participation of the conscious mind. Unlike a disease, which hits you when you are at your lowest ebb and your defenses are down, automatic behavior can hit you at any time. As a matter of fact, the healthier you are, the stronger your conditioned reflexes are.

As an example of automatic behavior, let us consider a tearful inmate. "I had it all Doc," he said. He had gotten out of prison on parole; he had gotten a good job; he was living happily with his children and their mother; he literally had money in his pocket. All was good. Until he entered a store with his children, got distracted and put some merchandise in his pocket (he used to shoplift regularly to support his past drug addiction). But now, bang. Back to jail with charges of shoplifting (minor) and violation of parole (major). The latter charge would send him back to prison for years. Hence the tears.

At a time when this man's attention was engaged, his automatic behavior kicked in and he shoplifted, more or less on autopilot. Technically he did not even relapse. With a substance relapse involved it is worse; because with a relapse, the substance itself feeds back to the complex reflex, causing the relapse to continue.

Beyond Addiction. Thankfully, substance dependence is not as much a disease as 12-step programs would have us believe. Economists point out that most addicts give up their addictions on their own in their 30's. (Think about it; what chronic disease can you just walk away from?) Clinically, it seems that other behaviors can take over from addiction behaviors. Economically, it seems that addicts are making the choice not to be addicts any more.

Whichever model is correct, it seems that addicts can outgrow their addictions.

They won't outgrow them, though, if "kindly" doctors diagnose them as "bipolar" and treat them chronically with addictive substances. The "kindly" doctors substitute legal drugs for illegal ones. The people remain addicts; but now their drugs come from doctors. And if they miss their legal drugs they may relapse into illegal ones.

This meddling by doctors is worse with methadone maintenance and now with buprenorphine maintenance. Funny thing: methadone has been available for decades. Yet the opiate overdose plague seems to be getting more pervasive.

Although some swear by it, methadone or buprenorphine maintenance continues a subject's dependence upon opiates. Even worse, the withdrawal and detox from either of these opiates is prolonged. And the fact that methadone and buprenorphine are drugs cushions a person from the slings and arrows of outrageous fortune, so that the opiate lifts the person's emotional weights; but the person does not get emotionally stronger. Add to that the morbid obesity and rotten teeth that so often accompany methadone treatment, and you wonder why anyone would keep addicts bound with their "golden handcuffs" (you will hear inmates call it that). But methadone clinics have a constant income with their methadone clients, and seem to have strong lobbyists in Congress. Buprenorphine is new, but has advocates as well.

A better treatment for alcoholism and opiate dependence is naltrexone. There are even some preliminary indications that this agent may be helpful in cocaine addiction. At the time of this writing the evidence for naltrexone use in cocaine dependence is only preliminary, but the medication has FDA indications for use in alcoholism and opiate dependence.

The way naltrexone works is simple: it takes the edge off the addict's craving; but this is not the main addiction-busting effect. The main effect is that naltrexone blocks the high. In theory and in practice, an addict cannot get high from his opiate or alcohol if he has sufficient naltrexone on board. That breaks the Crave-Seek-Find-Use cycle (see below). The addict drinks or shoots up, and the frenzy that often accompanies the approach to using the substance subsides. At that time the addict looks at himself and asks, "Why did I do that? That was stupid!"

See Appendix ME for more on naltrexone, but for now we note that it is sad that methadone is subsidized and provided free, continuing the addiction, while naltrexone—which ends an addiction—is not subsidized and must be paid for with the addict's insurance. Naltrexone is available as a daily pill, a three-month pellet—male addicts have been known to cut the pellet out in order to get high—and a monthly injection, which they are stuck with because they cannot cut it out.

Drugs vs Medications

As used here a drug is any substance which will have the same mind-altering effect, whether the subject is normal or has a mental illness. The benzodiazepines are drugs. Opiates, cocaine and marijuana are drugs. Quetiapine, hydroxyzine, gabapentin and topiramate are drugs. Gabapentin and topiramate in particular have been prescribed for "bipolar" disorder. But when their use has been investigated in randomized controlled trials, they have no effect in true bipolar disorder, strictly diagnosed. For psychiatric purposes, they are drugs.

BZD's are alcohol in a pill: they disinhibit the user (inmates call it "the felony pill"), mess with her memory (they also call it "the amnesia pill") and when she is dependent upon them, the withdrawal can cause all the shakes, seizures, hallucinosis and DT's that you can see in alcohol withdrawal. Truly, benzodiazepines are alcohol in a pill. Withdrawal from quetiapine causes opiate-like withdrawal symptoms. You may call it 'heroin in a pill.'

Drugs produce sedation or stimulation. Drugs "help" anybody. They help them to feel mellow or high. Even when a doctor prescribes it, even when a person takes it legally, this chemical is a drug. Inmates seek drugs. Think of buprenorphine, benzodiazepines, amphetamine, gabapentin, hydroxyzine, methadone and quetiapine. They are all drugs. All of them.

There are some chemicals that are medications in higher doses, like amitriptyline, doxepin, mirtazapine and trazodone. But in lower doses, they are still only drugs. If a chemical is used as a sleeping pill, for our purposes it is still a drug.

There are some chemicals that are medications for pain. Gabapentin, TCA's, venlafaxine and duloxetine have been used successfully for pain. But in a jail setting, a psychiatrist prescribes nothing for pain. If the inmate is to get something for pain she must receive it from the general medical doctor, not from the psychiatrist. Yes, it is often more efficient to prescribe one chemical for two purposes. But venlafaxine and duloxetine can be used only for psychiatric purposes by a psychiatrist in a jail. Either look into the legitimacy of prescribing any psychiatric med for this inmate or collaborate with the general medical prescriber on what chemicals the two of you will prescribe together.

Ideally, medications are chemicals used to treat mental illness. They are good for little else. Medications do not "help" people who do not have a mental illness. Think SSRI. Medications generally do not produce much or any sedation or stimulation. Inmates generally do not seek medications. They take them when they must, to relieve the symptoms of psychiatric illness. Most inmates seek drugs to relieve the discomfort of being incarcerated, by design an uncomfortable process.

Chlorpromazine and quetiapine have been used to "treat" the condition diagnosed as "bipolar disorder." Actually, chlorpromazine is a well-known but old treatment for ADHD. People with ADHD who take this drug often note how calm they feel, how able to concentrate. Yet fast-forward a few decades to see the same people with their cases of tardive dyskinesia. It's not pretty. Today they take quetiapine; often you see it taken for sleep. Methylphenidate would do as well and not produce deleterious side effects, but the doctors are busy treating "bipolar disorder."

Don't expect inmates to complain of side effects. A number of them experience the massive adipogenic aspect of quetiapine or olanzapine or risperidone and/or have diabetes and say nothing. But when their new obesity is observed they will say "Oh yeah" and remember that their weight gain commenced when they started the antipsychotic. But they would rather have the sedation than complain of a side effect.

Although it is not usually taken for its mind-altering properties, baclofen is best thought of as a drug for withdrawal purposes. Stopping baclofen suddenly can cause a withdrawal syndrome which resembles benzodiazepine or alcohol withdrawal, especially when baclofen was taken in conjunction with a drug in people who have been dependent on benzodiazepines.

Moving on from Addiction to Recovery

Between Addiction and Recovery there is a transitional stage when inmates go through three phases as they take leave of their substances.

Withdrawal (nominally a week)—the body reacts to not having its accustomed substance. Often vital signs are elevated.

Detox (nominally a month)—the brain reacts to not having its accustomed substance. Consider it the "screaming receptors" phase. Classical detoxification facilities last a month, because of the massive craving often seen during this phase. I used to observe alcoholics recover from their "depression" after about a month dry, without meds. Out from under the "alcohol shadow"—it takes a month—they spontaneously recovered from their "depression." This confirms the wisdom of making detox programs a month long.

Rehabilitation (nominally a year)—the addict is learning to live without drugs. His life is no longer cushioned by its accustomed substance. There is an exaggerated response to stimuli because the inmate is used to having the substance mute every stimulus. The individual has an exaggerated response to normal events. This emotional dysregulation is often termed "mood swings." Clinicians who accept these complaints at face value run the risk of diagnosing "bipolar disorder" inappropriately. As a good rule of thumb, you cannot diagnose bipolar disorder within a year of someone's using substances, illegal or legal. That's right: any drugs, legal or illegal, and you reset the clock on diagnosing bipolar disorder. The most you can do is diagnose "bipolar disorder" which is a useless diagnosis. Instead, note the emotional dysregulation or mood instability as a symptom, and note the date of last substance use.

Normally, inmates will be referred to you in the withdrawal or detox phases of their transition. Inmates typically are unhappy during all three phases, especially if the process is involuntary. But they are more desperate in the first two phases. They want some kind of substance to soothe them in the worst way. When they are not ready to take leave of their substances they will express distress—figuratively kicking and screaming all the way—unwilling to withdraw from, detox from or live without their substances. If the clinician gives in and assuages an inmate's discomfort at this stage, the clinician is only prolonging the process. Bad: if the clinician eases the withdrawal and detox phases, the inmates do not fully understand how bad the withdrawal and detox were, and are more likely to return to their substances. Worse: if the clinician uses quetiapine or olanzapine to do the assuaging, the inmate becomes dependent on a drug that produces a metabolic nightmare.

Here is where the utility of an SSRI comes to the fore: if an inmate is telling the truth and she really does have a psychiatric illness, treating it with a medication will help the sufferer. However, if an inmate is feigning an illness or talking of his distress when he has to do without his substances, then an SSRI does not "help" him. He throws it away in disgust.

Save a life. Do no harm. What could be better than that?

The Addiction Cycle

Addiction follows a cycle.

Crave First, the addict has a trigger for his craving. This may be the craving itself, or something reminiscent of the addict life that produces a craving. Or it may be some circumstance the addict cannot cope with, so she craves her drug to help her cope. A simple rejection, for example, might dishearten an addict who is not accustomed to coping with rejection. So the addict looks for a bottle, a blunt or a needle. The complex conditioned reaction has been triggered.

Seek At the next stage the addict will seek a substance. This is automatic behavior, no matter how conscious the behavior seems to the addict or to observers.

Find At the next stage the addict will find the substance. There may be a further stage of learned behavior as the addict prepares the substance for use. Cooking up heroin or opening a bottle fall into this stage. Tension builds as the addict prepares for the next step. Where there is no preparation step the tension builds while the addict is searching for the substance.

Use The addict then will use the substance. This immediately relieves the tension that has built up as the addict has prepared to use the substance. The sensation of relief and the actions of the substance combine to alleviate the trigger and the craving.

Of course use of the substance induces a craving of its own which goes on to trigger another addiction cycle.

The Addict Cycle: Crave, Seek, Find, Use. That's about as basic a cycle as it gets.

Withdrawal

This is a medical process. It is often a medical emergency, involving seizures, out-of-control vital signs, sweating, nausea, etc. A whole expertise has arisen around withdrawal from alcohol and drugs. It involves nurses taking vital signs, assuring hydration and administering drugs. A psychiatrist will quickly find herself over her head. Withdrawal is best left to medical specialists. It may last one to two weeks.

Yes, in older times psychiatrists did manage withdrawal. Since most withdrawal is mild, patients did not get into too much trouble. But with severe withdrawal medical intervention is needed, often on an emergent basis. Again, the whole process is best left to medical specialists.

There is an exception. When psychiatrists have subspecialized in treating substances, they can develop an expertise in withdrawal. They may come to know more about how to manage withdrawal cases than medical specialists. In such cases, you might turn over the job to one of them.

Detox

The detoxification phase begins when withdrawal ends. Generally, a detox unit will not take a person who is still in withdrawal, still getting drugs to ease her way down.

The inmate might be grateful when the state has "saved my life" by pulling him from his drugs. Occasionally we do see this response. But more normally the withdrawal was involuntary, so the inmate comes to you seeking relief from his screaming receptors.

The key here is to determine whether the inmate was more or less well when he began his substances, or was suffering from a pre-existing psychiatric illness. This can be difficult, since substances can produce an illness. There is an 'alcohol shadow' that extends for about a month after stopping alcohol. A person is depressed from drinking and remains so while he is still under the alcohol shadow. Yet his depression will often lift after a month of sobriety even without any chemical intervention.

Recent research shows that continued exposure to opiates—even prescribed opiates—results in depression. Getting clean on coming into a jail can relieve this. This is one of many reasons not to continue methadone when a person enters a jail. (It is also true for psychiatric hospitals, but that is another story.)

If an inmate was not getting psychiatric care before coming to jail; if she was not even seeking psychiatric care before coming to jail, the decision is fairly easy: she might improve without chemical intervention once the detox phase has passed. Yet inmates—especially female inmates, who can be especially dramatic—often demand medications. They can be insistent in their demands. Of course they are looking for drugs, which you will not prescribe. But in cases where you are not sure if someone should get meds or not, go ahead and prescribe SSRI's or buspirone. Just stay away from drugs or "comfort pills" (anti-psychotics can be used this way, so beware).

Again: the SSRI's and buspirone treat mental illness without providing drug-like effects. If it reaches the inmate it will help in a week or three. If it does not provide the instant relief the inmate was looking for, she will stop the meds. You can then discontinue the med orders and drop the person from your census.

Avoid using gabapentin. See in Chapter 7 "What Not to Use For Depression." Bottom line: gabapentin potentiates substance abuse. See also Appendix ME.

Rehabilitation

The key here is to determine whether the inmate was more or less well when he began his substances, or was suffering from an abusive childhood. An inmate who was essentially "trapped" by substance use generally needs to get "clean" or "dry;" he can take it from there. An inmate whose substance abuse was part of a lifetime of dysfunction will need ongoing psycho-therapy support; in a word, rehabilitation. Inter-ventions here include DBT, resiliency training, assertiveness training, anger management, EMDR—all outside the purview of psychiatry as normally practiced in jails. Maybe the inmate needs an SSRI for depressive symptoms, maybe not. Rehabilitation is psychosocial, not psychiatric.

There is a concept known as PAWS, or the Post-Acute Withdrawal Syndrome. PAWS results in a roller coaster of symptoms, and often in-volves intense craving. Research has shown that craving peaks at about six months. It's a broad average, though, so expect to see craving at any time during the rehab phase.

The advantage of a correctional environment: an inmate cannot just walk off a unit to pre-maturely end therapy. Of course, drugs can be obtained in most jails and prisons, but the consequences on discovery can be severe.

Maintenance and Long Term Rehabilitation

The first word on maintenance of abstinence or sobriety was "One Day at a Time" from AA. I will never forget talking to a man who was crisply attired in a business suit, ready to go out after lunch and greet financiers. He told me he had been sober for 17 years. Over the entire time he said alcohol had exerted a constant pull. Staying sober had been "one day at a time" for him.

That was before naltrexone. In those days, we had only disulfiram, which would give you nausea if you drank.

Today we still have AA and NA, with their group support of the abstinence process. There are more clinics now. Hopefully, people who are hurting can get group and individual psychotherapy from mental health providers.

You expect addicts to relapse at least once during detox or rehab. The key will be preventing an ongoing or a recurrent relapse. Breaking the addict cycle is important. Stopping the addiction without something more, basically freezes the inmate at the craving stage. He remains uncomfortable in his desire for the substance. Breaking the addict cycle allows him to move out of the cycle and on to other patterns in life.

To facilitate what could be considered an augmented abstinence, we physicians can provide naltrexone, which derails the addict cycle at the *use* phase. It prevents the expected response (relief of tension) and pushes the addict up into a meta- or observing phase. Ideally the tension will get lost in the addict's realization that he was in the middle of a relapse. The addict will shift from a thoughtless execution of a conditioned reflex to a thoughtful contemplation of his addiction behavior.

This is far superior to the substitute addiction model, where the doctor provides the addict with a legal substitute for an illegal drug. That model merely prolongs the addict's addiction. Substitute addiction has not prevented whole swaths of people from getting addicted to heroin and dying from overdoses of heroin and unknown amounts of fentanyl or carfentanyl.

Perhaps this was the best we could do in the past: provide time for the addict to change his thinking, detoxify and walk away from his addiction. But with the availability of naltrexone, we have an alternative form of treatment for the addiction.

Rehabilitation from addiction can also occur in the context of long-term incarceration. Here the inmate is faced with increased cost and increased sanctions involved in acquiring the addictive substance. Usually such long-term incarceration is found in prisons. But sometimes inmates stay in jails for years. In such cases, physicians can encourage new ways of thinking about alcohol and drug use. Mental health counselors can encourage adaptive coping in the face of stressors. Importantly, inmates must come to believe that change is possible.

Bottom line: the involved psychiatrist must support rehabilitation from substance abuse with appropriate prescribing. We should not enable continued substance abuse by prescribing drugs which encourage addictive behavior.

Self-Management And Recovery Training (SMART)

This is also called HARP, for Health And Recovery Peer program. These are forms of cognitive-behavior therapy programs aimed at substance abusing populations. The "self-management" parts of the names of these therapies calls to mind DBT, aimed at people with borderline personality disorder. The similarity may not be accidental. In any case, these are growing programs which may find a place at your jails. Any help will be welcome.

Chapter 7
Treatment with Medication

Treating inmates in a jail is different from treating patients in a hospital and very different from treating patients in your outpatient practice. For one thing, you don't have to please them to keep their business. They are looking for help. They can't get out of jail, or they would not be seeing you. There is not some other doctor where they will turn to get their comfort pills.

Your first rule: Don't work to please an inmate.

An inmate may complain of "anxiety." An inmate may complain of trouble sleeping; of ADHD symptoms. Inmates come to you requesting comfort pills. They may be very disappointed when they learn that we do not treat insomnia or ADHD. We may treat anxiety as a part of a depressive illness, but we don't treat anxiety *per se*. Our job is to treat mental illness, not simply make inmates more comfortable.

You may be familiar with the practices of detox programs because they, like jail programs, take people off drugs. But detox programs exist to make their patients comfortable as they come off their substances. This is how they keep their patients. Seen from an addiction perspective, making patients comfortable is one of the great mistakes detox programs make: patients leave programs still craving their substances because they are not fully detoxified. Worse, their automatic behavior has not been addressed. Jails in general are the best detox programs because they do not make inmates comfortable. Inmates are fully detoxed if they stay long enough. And they learn to cope with circumstances without substances, which can break the addiction cycle.

We do not give chemicals to people who are not mentally ill

Inmates are in jail. They are locked up. They *should* feel anxious. They *should* feel upset. The fact that they are not sleeping is a normal response to adverse circumstances or detox, not a symptom of a mental illness. ICD-10 even has a code for this—Z65.1. A Z-code in ICD-10 is outside of psychiatric disorders.

Some people will not be satisfied

They don't want to cope with their lives. You will end up treating their "anxiety," their dysphoria, their inability to cope with stressful circumstances. And these are the inmates who are normal people.

For most of the inmates you see, you are dealing with people who have had a depressive neurosis most of their lives. If you keep giving them drugs like diphenhydramine or hydroxyzine, they will "improve" for a time, but then they come back to you complaining of more anxiety. Whenever something bad happens, they need "a little something" to help them get through their reactions.

Inmates are not children. They can cope with the bad things that come with life. But when bad things happen they want to have "something to get by," something to help them "cope." Pretty soon they need "something" to help them "cope" and "get by" every day. Thus if you chase symptoms you will never catch up.

So: Don't chase symptoms

Now this may seem to violate the whole approach of modern medicine where you monitor symptoms, note as symptoms disappear and fashion your treatment accordingly. If you practice with an eye on reviewers and managed care, you may reflexively keep track of individual symptoms. But that approach was never formulated with liars in mind. So go ahead and record the symptoms and let the symptoms guide your treatment (you will also pay attention to signs) but don't let the 'symptoms' *drive* the treatment.

Always remember: Inmates lie

Inmates are often criminals who spend their whole lives working to con things out of people so they don't have to work for those things. They have spent years and decades learning to lie convincingly. Since you don't spend all your life learning how to pick out liars and their lies, you are not as good at picking up prevarications as inmates are in making up falsehoods. So always take reported symptoms with a grain of salt.

You have to dance on the line. Inmates report symptoms, and symptoms are the core of illness. But who better than a psychiatrist to parse the need for meds within an inmate's complaints, versus his requests for drugs?

Use a medication, not a drug

In general, you treat a person according to the mental illness that appears to be present. With inmates in particular, let them lie if they want to. You won't know it anyway. If an inmate complains of anxiety and depression, you use an SSRI. When inmates have been lying to you in the hopes of getting drugs prescribed to them, they are disappointed. Often they simply drop treatment. When they learn that repeated visits result in their receiving non-drug medications, they will give it up. They will drop off your census, leaving you with more time that you can devote to the inmates who really need your help.

If you want to increase your workload, medicate the symptoms with drugs. I knew one psychiatrist who prescribed two weeks of hydroxyzine every time she saw an inmate. This is like the pediatrician who gives lollipops to children who come to see him. The kids return to get more.

I know another psychiatrist who chases symptoms. His inmates are always complaining and he is always racking his brain, trying to think of chemicals that will not disappoint his inmates. He will not understand that his inmates have an infinite reservoir of complaints. They are always looking to get more drugs. His inmate load is larger than he can service. He is always inundated with overwork.

Neither she nor he have any time for truly needy inmates, inmates who may have recondite illnesses and actually need their doctor's expertise in finding and treating their mental illnesses.

You can't treat everything with chemicals

The VA has been working for 50 years to find a medication that will treat PTSD. The fact that they are still looking should tell you something. More particularly, antipsychotics do not work on the primary symptoms of PTSD. The side effects of antipsychotics may reduce the intensity of the PTSD symptoms, but to gain that reduced intensity, you are exposing the inmate to the risks of diabetes, obesity and other life-shortening problems.

People who suffer psychological injury need psychological treatment. We do not yet have successful medication treatments for PTSD, dysthymia, or BPD. We do have drugs and medications that reduce the impact of those disorders, but never kid yourself into thinking that any physical intervention will cure any of those illnesses. For example, people with abusive backgrounds and other adverse childhood events do not respond well to ECT.

Some children grow up in families where they are always belittled and put down. They may be molested or become the target of violence at unexpected times and places, seemingly at every turn. They grow up expecting unhappiness and abuse everywhere they go. They expect to be hit at any moment, with no warning. There are people who whenever they encounter a group of people, think that members of the group are talking about them and putting them down. And yet some psychiatrists have tried ECT on people with such issues; the effects are temporary or minimal. SSRI's have their positive effects on these issues, but you should temper your expectations. Cures come with psychotherapy and time.

Specialists in personality disorder describe people who are hypersensitive, who have mood changes and who can experience voices, especially at night. They also note that these patients do not respond well to medications. This was well known in the past. It is still true today.

When you begin to realize that you can't cure everything with chemicals, you are ready to receive the wisdom of Harry Callahan in the movie Magnum Force:

"A man's got to know his limitations."

Before you go making sardonic jokes, know that it is true for women as well. It is also a lesson for inmates.

In this day of miracle medications, the idea that not every condition can be treated with a pill can seem foreign to an inmate. After all, they are used to fending off all feelings with drugs; and benzodiazepines can reduce both anxiety and fear. Why can't you fix their bad feelings right now? Why can't you ease their detox discomfort right away? Why must they wait one to two weeks to find out if your antidepressant pill will help them? But one can get some help for PTSD, dysphoria and social phobia with an SSRI or an SNRI if one is willing to wait for it. If you do not use drugs, inmates have no choice but to wait for the medication to help them, and to control themselves in the interim.

You can begin to realize what damage chemicals can do, whether we call them 'drugs' or 'medicines,' if you consider that before they used stimulants widely for ADHD, doctors 'treated' agitated children with thioridazine, chlorpromazine and stronger antipsychotics (today they use quetiapine). Before doctors considered that children might be showing a reaction formation to the abuse they were suffering, or a traumatic event the child had experienced, they simply tried to snuff the agitation with an antipsychotic. The side effect of those chemicals was sedation and the children were duly sedated. Because non-psychotic patients are more likely to develop tardive dyskinesia than psychotic patients, these medicated and sedated children sometimes developed TD as they got older. Today, of course, we psychiatrists are so much more sophisticated. We call the children "bipolar" and treat them with chemicals like quetiapine, risperidone, divalproex and olanzapine; we make them obese and watch them develop diabetes. Not to mention that early exposure to antipsychotics causes dysthymia later in life. Such progress.

Some Limiting Principles

To make it easier to defend yourself in court, always use medications on-label. Avoid off-label uses. Do not claim that gabapentin and topiramate have any use in bipolar disorder, for example. In randomized controlled trials in genuine bipolar disorder, they have failed. There is a reason they have not earned a psychiatric indication. They were invented for seizure control, and have been found useful for reducing neuropathic pain and for preventing migraine headaches. These are nonpsychiatric indications.

In fact, *avoid trivial uses for major meds like antipsychotics.* An inmate may exercise bad judgment and allow you to prescribe risperidone for anxiety or olanzapine for sleep. The companies that make them may even have obtained indications to use antipsychotic meds for purposes other than controlling psychosis. But judges and juries will take a dim view of such poor thinking, thinking that leads unsuspecting patients to suffer diabetes, dyslipidemia and obesity, not to mention gynecomastia. Inmates can survive the nervousness they call "anxiety." They can survive initial insomnia. They might have a harder time surviving a metabolic syndrome or dementia. Don't use these heavy-duty meds for trivial reasons.

Results of Non-Treatment

Leaving anxiety and ADHD and insomnia untreated will not result in catastrophe. Inmates will complain but if they have anxiety and ADHD, they can develop the skills to cope. If they have insomnia, they can learn sleep hygiene. For one thing, they have to get up early to take their meds. If they stay up all day, and do this day after day, they will start getting tired at night, tired enough to sleep.

In jails we should prescribe medications, not drugs. We treat mental illness, not normal responses to unhappy situations—no PRN's. We need to know our limitations. And above all, we must strive to do no harm.

ADHD

There are people who cannot sit still, cannot pay attention, do things suddenly without thinking first (impulsivity), and complain of not being able to get to sleep at night, staying up with "racing thoughts." They may show easy distractibility, and complain of poor memory (they complain that they cannot pay attention when others speak). These people, of course, have ADHD.

Funny thing, though: when a psychiatrist hears ADHD symptoms he/she usually diagnoses "bipolar" disorder, blowing off early childhood experiences. Family Practice doctors usually hear the ADHD and diagnose correctly.

You don't usually treat ADHD in an adult jail, because ADHD does not usually prevent an inmate from living in jail. However, if Custody complains of an inmate's behavior, it may be from ADHD. Then you can consider lithium, which helps in ADHD. If you prescribe more than 300mg BID you will see no improvement, and maybe some side effects. If your jail has not banned bupropion because inmates abuse it (they snort it), it can be an effective treatment for ADHD. Buspirone occasionally helps ADHD, as can venlafaxine.

Treating Depression and Anxiety

Inmates who describe a depressive syndrome ought to be treated. Although they might be asking for drugs, they will generally accept medications. Unlike TCA's, SSRI's will treat both major depression and dysthymia. Because SSRI's do nothing for an inmate if she is not mentally ill, inmates will not malinger to receive SSRI's. Word gets around, and when it becomes known that an inmate cannot get a drug from you, inmates will stop pestering you and leave the field clear for those that want or need medication.

Inmates may complain of "anxiety." Unpack that. The inmate may complain that he can't sit still, can't sleep and does things impulsively. This, of course, is ADHD mislabeled as "anxiety." If an inmate complains that he is afraid because he is here, maybe he has fear, not anxiety. Think about it: your inmate is held captive in a concrete box, surrounded by criminals. He should be afraid, or he is in his element.

Feel free to treat the inmate's anxiety and depression with buspirone and all the different SSRI's and SNRI's until the inmate has tried them all. Then tell the inmate she has exhausted all the options; there is nothing left to treat her with. Actually, she was just fishing for a benzodiazepine or a "legal" drug like hydroxyzine. After she knows there is no pill left, she can get busy in therapy, if the anxiety or depression is genuine, or abandon the pursuit of drugs if the symptoms were fake.

Buspirone might be useful for anxiety, but it will not reduce panic attacks. That requires counseling, and perhaps an antidepressant.

What Not to Use for Depression and Anxiety

Avoid all TCA's, even when the inmate is specifically asking for doxepin. They can be used as sleeping pills or anxiolytics. Even though a TCA is often a medication that can help, some inmates will hoard it, looking to get high or get a "really good sleep." An overdose of a TCA—including doxepin—can kill. So *don't use a TCA*.

Bupropion can treat depression. But it is also used to treat ADHD, which we do not treat in jails.

Bupropion can be crushed and snorted to get an amphetamine-like high. This chemical is forbidden in some jails. In others, it is crushed and smothered in water to inhibit diversion. Where bupropion is crushed or available only in the immediate release form, *do not prescribe more than 150mg per dose* because of the risk of *seizures*. If an inmate was taking larger doses on the outside, he was taking it in the CR or XL forms (we hope).

Gabapentin and **Topiramate** are *drugs*. In the hands of medical specialists they are medications for seizures, pain or migraines. But these are things that nonpsychiatric doctors treat, not psychiatrists. They are not "mood stabilizers," any more than diazepam is. Every time they have been tried for actual bipolar cases, rigorously diagnosed, they have failed. For psychiatry, they are drugs. *Do not prescribe either in a jail.*

Mirtazapine and **Trazodone** seem safe for an inmate to use, but there is a market for them wherever they are prescribed. Both are soporific. They are sleeping pills, especially in smaller doses. Mirtazapine 15mg or trazodone 50-100mg are sleep aids, and will not treat depression. Larger doses can be split and sold in pieces. Both are drugs inmates seek, even when they do not have a mental illness. In facilities where they have been discontinued for all inmates, a number of inmates stopped asking for psych meds when they could no longer get one or the other specific drug. These meds are easily diverted to the underground drug market and should not be used. *Do not prescribe either in a jail.*

Hydroxyzine is a drug. It has no psychiatric indication. Some psychiatrists swear by its anxiolytic properties. But it has long been used to extend the effects of opiates in postop patients, who in general are not mentally ill. It is not a treatment for mental illness: it is not a psychiatric medication. It is a drug. *Do not prescribe it in a jail.*

Antipsychotics Some practitioners prescribe antipsychotics for anxiety and/or depression, in essence evading the prohibition against benzodiazepines. This is bad practice: you are using the antipsychotic for its sedating property, which is a side effect. People with anxiety and depression are not psychotic, and should not be exposed to the other actual and potential side effects of antipsychotic drugs simply because a practitioner wants to "help." First of all we must do no harm. *Do not prescribe one in a jail* unless the inmate is truly psychotic.

Some practitioners chafe under the restriction of eschewing a benzodiazepine in a jail. They want to use gabapentin, hydroxyzine, topiramate or an antipsychotic to "treat" an inmate's "anxiety." More likely, they are reducing an inmate's discomfort of being in a jail without his or her accustomed drugs. Don't fall into this trap. Benzodiazepines are forbidden for good reasons. Don't try to go around the restriction. Don't do it.

New information on gabapentin. In 2018, NJ practitioners received the following email: "Effective May 7, 2018, the New Jersey Division of

Consumer Affairs . . . require New Jersey licensed pharmacies and registered out-of-State pharmacies to electronically transmit information to the Division about prescriptions dispensed for gabapentin. The recognition of gabapentin as a "drug of concern" stems from national prescription and overdose data. New Jersey is joining a growing list of states who have already begun to monitor gabapentin use, including those that have scheduled the medication at the state level.

"Studies have shown that gabapentin prescribing in the United States has increased 49% over the past five years resulting in 64 million prescription dispensations in 2016. Additionally, the prevalence of gabapentin abuse in the general population is only 1.2%, but increases to a staggering 15% - 22% amongst opioid users; likely a direct result of the potentiating effects caused by combination therapy. In New Jersey, over the past two years, the presence of gabapentin in post-mortem toxicology reports increased by more than 1,000% overall and by more than 3,000% in the opioid-use subgroup."

In other words, do not prescribe the stuff.

Specific Guidelines for Treating Depression

Start with an SSRI like citalopram (20-40mg/d), fluoxetine (20-60mg/d) or sertraline

(50-200mg/d). Start with a half dose for a few days to minimize the risk of side effects.

Don't expect that SSRI's will help someone who is in detox—someone who has not gone a month without drugs of abuse and withdrawal drugs like chlordiazepoxide. In fact, sometimes allowing an inmate to finish the detox period will be enough to resolve a "depression," with no meds needed. But don't expect results in two weeks if the inmate is still in detox.

If your first SSRI does not help an inmate to feel better, she can try another SSRI. After that, consider an SNRI. But remember: sometimes dysthymia does not respond to medications. Adjunctive antipsychotics should be avoided, unless the inmate has been psychotic. Hallucinations during withdrawal and detox are not a reason to start antipsychotics.

Treating Catatonia

When someone looks catatonic, you must first determine if the cause is medical. If so, medical people should deal with the situation. But if the inmate has catatonia, it is still a medical emergency. Catatonics die. It doesn't matter if the underlying cause is schizophrenia, a manic episode or an organic psychosis; you can't manage it in a jail. So if the inmate is truly catatonic, get the person out to an emergency room. You can worry about the underlying diagnosis later.

If you are unfortunate enough to practice in a situation where it is impossible to get an inmate immediate medical attention, you might have to treat a catatonic. If so, treat the catatonia with lorazepam in addition to the antipsychotic. Lorazepam is a specific treatment for catatonia. Alprazolam, clonazepam or any other benzodiazepine will not do. Clinical experience demonstrates that lorazepam IM followed by lorazepam PO is likely to help bring an inmate back from catatonia. Whether you can discontinue the lorazepam later, is an issue for later. But first of all and last of all, try to get the catatonic inmate to a physical hospital.

Treating Psychosis

When an inmate has a withdrawal psychosis, it is best not to treat anything except the withdrawal, and the medical specialist is in charge of that. When an inmate hears voices as part of a PTSD, the voices may be intrapsychic voices. Such voices often do not respond to antipsychotics, since they are not part of a psychotic process (but see below). When a grieving inmate hears voices, he usually attributes them to the people he has lost in his life. The psychiatrist should take care in treating such phenomena. Sometimes an antipsychotic actually helps, but the psychiatrist should ponder the case before pulling out the prescription pad.

When you have a legitimate psychosis, it is time for an antipsychotic medication. An illegal drug-induced psychosis generally responds better to low potency meds like chlorpromazine, than to high potency meds like fluphenazine. Yet because so many inmates pursue chlorpromazine for general sedation, the history which might support the use of chlorpromazine will be highly suspect. Treating a drug-induced psychosis with AM haloperidol or risperidone will help you avoid inmates who are seeking sedation and lying to you about their voices.

Otherwise, with a psychotic mania or schizo-phrenia, you treat the psychosis as you normally would. However, remember that often people are just as satisfied with first-generation antipsych-otic meds as they are with second-generation meds. While inmates can be uncomfortable with the side effects of first-generation antipsychotics, the second-generation antipsychotics can cause diabetes, morbid obesity and dyslipidemia, medic-al millstones which physically harm the inmate forever, long decades after the therapy has stopped (we recently had such a case). Diabetes, for example, makes dementia more likely. Take great care before you consider prescribing one of these medications.

Finally, in managing people with psychosis, recall that they may be less responsive to the prospect of rewards than nonpsychotic people. There is recent research that suggests a neural reason for this, but in general when you look at decades of description and research, you see constant themes of blunting, lack of motivation and impaired responsiveness to normal life events. Keep these factors in mind when you discuss managing psychotic inmates with Custody.

Schizophrenia—Delayed Relapse

Back in the 1950's, when psychiatrists were first treating schizophrenia with antipsychotics, they would stop treating patients with antipsychotics as soon as the psychoses stopped. Patients would remain well without meds for a variable length of time, up to a year. But a majority would relapse into psychosis. This was the origin of the "maintenance dose" of antipsychotics in psychiatric practice. During this med-free interval, patients would look good, since the side effects of antipsychotics fade rapidly, while the psychotogenic effects of doing without meds show up much more slowly. For this reason, do not allow yourself to fall into the "false good" trap. If your patient remains well without meds, this is good. But always be prepared to restart them. And always be amenable to providing such inmates with a maintenance dose. Any antipsychotic— even 1mg/day—is better than nothing.

We try to get patients to use depot injections of antipsychotic medications. We are also involved in confidentiality. But I wonder if injections given in a group setting would encourage patients to accept IM meds. There might be a camaraderie to the process.

PTSD

Often the inmate with PTSD does not know that she has PTSD. It may be cloaked in her substance abuse or it may be labeled as "bipolar." Her problems may be laid to "anxiety" and "depression." Even our colleagues blithely treat the symptoms with chemicals, as if the person came to them with an unremarkable history and simply developed depression and/or anxiety. But you know by now that you have to look at an inmate's whole history. Often the depression, anxiety and social phobia stem from past history or an incident that immediately preceded the symptoms. When you routinely take whole life histories from people you will be amazed at how often inmates and their doctors ignore traumatic events to diagnose mere anxiety and depression or call it "bipolar."

PTSD is a psychological injury and requires psychological treatment like EMDR or the FDA-approved device for PTSD (for a possible exception, see below). If an inmate also has depression and anxiety, treat those. But don't imagine that you are treating all of the inmate's problems with your chemicals. You're not. And the inmate has to know this. She is used to other chemicals—drugs—which cover up the symptom as long as the person is intoxicated. But drugs, even marijuana, leave the underlying disorder untouched. This is why you must educate the patient and either provide her with the therapy she needs while she is incarcerated, or provide her with the information she needs to acquire appropriate therapy when she is released from jail.

If the inmate complains of *nightmares* at least she is saying she *sleeps at night*. Some inmates are not smart enough to know that complaints of not sleeping are not compatible with complaints of nightmares, which necessarily must occur during sleep. In such a case, the complaints of sleeplessness and nightmares may be contra-factual and both may be outright lies. If an inmate complains that she is afraid to fall asleep because of the trauma-related nightmares that accompany her sleep, this sounds like a legitimate history. But remember that since the 1960's it has been observed that successful treatment with antidepressants has been associated with "vivid dreams," often nightmares. These nightmares are generally not the inmate re-experiencing past events.

Although prazosin is widely used to suppress trauma-related nightmares, some randomized controlled trials have failed to show benefits in VA studies of PTSD. So maybe it is helpful, maybe not. Hypotension is a problem for those who take this. And it may not be on your formulary.

Clonidine is sometimes used as a substitute for prazosin, but it does not work. There are some people with ADHD who feel calmer on clonidine, but this is the only benefit for those with nightmares.

Some practitioners prescribe antipsychotics for nightmares. In general, this is bad practice: you are using the antipsychotic for its sedating property, which is a side effect. And if you don't put the person to sleep, the antipsychotic med does not stop the nightmares. People with PTSD are usually not psychotic (but see below) and should not be exposed to the other actual and potential side effects of antipsychotic drugs simply because a practitioner wants to "help." First of all we must do no harm.

Note: **the VA no longer recommends any drugs or medications** as a first-line treatment for PTSD.

Inmates with PTSD can be treated with antidepressants for any depressive symptoms, as well as for anxiety. SSRI's are helpful and sertraline, in particular, has been associated with positive responses in PTSD. Buspirone can treat anxiety, and venlafaxine has been approved for social phobia. However, the inmate must not expect too much from pills. Cognitive therapy and individual therapy have had good results, especially EMDR; recently, the FDA approved a device to treat PTSD. This makes sense: PTSD is a psychological injury and requires psychological treatment. Inmates can also be counseled on coping with nightmares. This will be covered in the chapter on counseling.

Recent genome-wide association studies have found some overlap between people suffering from schizophrenia and people suffering from PTSD and auditory hallucinations. Some cases of schizophrenia see their first symptoms during or after a trauma or stress. There used to be an 'immigrant syndrome,' for example. And psychiatrists who work in basic training posts are familiar with people who 'crack up' in training. So it may be rational to treat voices in PTSD with antipsychotics. But be careful. Sometimes people experience 'visitations' of persons they once knew. This is a phenomenon long recognized (centuries) to be associated with grief, and is not something that needs to be treated. In general, it requires all your expertise to figure out whether to treat or not to treat PTSD voices with antipsychotic meds. You will be wrong sometimes, but we are dealing with human beings and a difficult illness. Tread carefully. Starting treatment with an antidepressant (SSRI's, SNRI's or—in your practices outside jails—TCA's like doxepin) and you might see a resolution of the voices, without need to involve an antipsychotic, with all of its baggage. Take care.

Note: MDMA (ecstasy) is in Phase III trials for PTSD. But because it is a drug of abuse, expect inmates to want it. If it is approved, we can expect all the false allegations of PTSD that we used to see, and for the same reason—to get drugs.

Tourette's—med or psych?

Tourette's Disorder carries a psychiatric coding number in both ICD-9 and ICD-10: 307.23 and F95.2. It is a tic disorder, and tics might seem physical. ICD-9 has them in sort of a miscellaneous psychiatric category, as does ICD-10. So it is categorized as a psychiatric condition.

Tourette's has been treated with haloperidol and pimozide, both first-generation antipsychotics. More recently, clonidine has been found to be helpful. Other treatments are available, but will not be covered here.

RLS—med or psych?

Restless Leg Syndrome is a neurologic syndrome where the sufferer has odd sensations in the affected parts of his body—most often the legs, but it can be anywhere—and the irresistible urge to move the affected area or limb. It can be very uncomfortable, and can keep the patient awake. Because it is not a psychiatric condition, RLS belongs to your GP to treat. So why are we covering it here?

Some medical specialists consider this to be psychiatric. Why do they think that? One reason is the RLS has a strong overlap with ADHD. Another reason is the resemblance of RLS to akathisia, which is a side effect of antipsychotic medications, especially first-generation antipsychotics. Akathisia can sometimes be difficult to distinguish from RLS, but the physical discomfort that plagues RLS sufferers is not part of the akathisia symptom complex.

The main feeling in RLS is the "creepy crawly" sensation inside the thigh muscles of the suffering person. The thigh is the most common site. Any place is vulnerable to a crawling or painful feeling inside the afflicted part. This condition may wait to ambush a person by starting as soon as he relaxes or lies down.

ADHD generally makes people restless, but without the odd sensations that build up in the RLS sufferer. Both conditions can cause a worsening of symptoms as the person relaxes but in ADHD, the whole person is restless; where in RLS there is a portion of the body that has sensations and must be moved.

Akathisia is motor restlessness. In the words of an old song "You can't sit down. You can't sit down. You got to move move move around and round." Akathisia is Greek for not sitting. It can cause immense suffering. When combined with akinesia (psychic paralysis) it can be excruciating. Some people have become suicidal when an antipsychotic or SSRI causes akathisia. Second-generation antipsychotics, though they don't cause pseudoparkinsonism as often as first-generation antipsychotics, cause plenty of akathisia. If you are not careful, you may mistake it for anxiety or some other subjective complaint. Again, it differs from RLS in that you do not hear inmates complaining of the physical symptoms.

When inmates have RLS, refer them to your medical specialist. When an inmate has akathisia, you can try changing the offending medication. Or you can try treating him with propranolol, diphenhydramine or hydroxyzine. Often amantadine is useful for treating akathisia and akinesia.

Treating Neurologic Conditions

Why is this here? Shouldn't your GP treat seizures and other neurologic conditions? It is true that GP's treat outright seizures, but sometimes psychiatrists run into conditions that blur the line.

ND-PAE. According to the head of NIAAA, crack addicts ("crack-heads") drink to buffer their crack use. According to research, the damage done to pregnant women's fetuses was from the alcohol, not the crack (personal communication). The helpless children were referred to as "crack babies." Now that it is known they have ND-PAE (F88) or Fetal Alcohol Spectrum Disorder (FASD, Q86 in ICD-10) or even full-blown Fetal Alcohol Syndrome (FAS, or Q86 in ICD-10) how do you treat it?

Well, you can try carbamazepine 200mg BID or more. Raise the doses only after getting CBZ levels, and remember that using carbamazepine with fluoxetine can be problematic. Recall also that people with an east Asian heritage are known to have an increased risk of SJS with CBZ. Be careful.

People with irritability may respond to an SSRI or buspirone. Sometimes divalproex is a useful alternative to carbamazepine.

As for the low IQ that is frequently a part of ND-PAE, you can't make someone smarter by giving them meds.

TLD. Temporolimbic Dysfunction can be tricky to diagnose. People with this problem often hear voices or music from earliest childhood. Current symptoms include out-of-place smells (they smell something burning or sweet when everyone should smell of body odor and feces), frequent déjà vu (to minimize faking, ask "Do you have a lot of déjà vu, a little déjà vu or *no* déjà vu?"), and emotional instability.

The treatment for TLD will be disappointing for the drug-seeking inmate: carbamazepine. Again, raise doses only after getting blood levels. Sometimes divalproex is a useful alternative to carbamazepine. Be careful with CBZ.

The condition differs from schizophrenia in the sufferers are not autistic at all, the way schizophrenics would be. When they respond to anticonvulsants, you know they have been spared from a lifetime of suffering . . . from psychiatric meds.

TBI. People who have experienced traumatic brain injuries sometimes know they have been damaged, sometimes not. Again, the treatments will be carbamazepine and sometimes divalproex.

The No-PRN Rule

Don't use PRN meds. Yes, in a prison or an emergency department you may have to, but a jail is neither of those. You are far more likely to get someone who is acting out so that you will administer a PRN.

If an inmate is having a panic attack with all the drama involved you administer an IM dose of lorazepam, right? Wrong! Clip on a pulse oximeter and show the agitated person that she has fully saturated her blood with O2. Then you let her cool down over the next 15-30 minutes or so. She will do that. After she has cooled down, you or some other medical person can point out to her that she did not die, that she can weather this adrenaline storm. If she can learn the lesson, it will make her stronger and better able to resist her next panic attack. By the way, sometimes people experience muscle cramping. This is due to hyperventilating and it will fade as the blood pH normalizes.

Labs

Clinically, the purpose of a blood level is to make sure a person is not running too high a level of a substance. If the level is theoretically low, you should not care as long as your patient is getting well. We treat people, not lab tests.

You should track renal functions quarterly if you are treating with lithium. If you are treating someone with a second-generation antipsychotic, you should get monthly weights. You should also keep track of hemoglobin A1c, lipid profiles and prolactin levels. Follow the latest official guidelines for treatment.

Cautions

First-generation antipsychotics

When you are treating inmates with first-generation antipsychotics, you must guard against not only extrapyramidal system side effects but also tardive dyskinesia. Look for pseudoparkinsonism, dystonia, akathisia and akinesia. Also, in your mental status exams, remark on the presence or absence of buccal-lingual movements or the presence of other components of TD. Remember that some call these neurotoxic chemicals.

Second-generation antipsychotics

When you are treating inmates with second-generation antipsychotics, recall a number of side effects. First of all, they may cause diabetes. Separately from diabetes, they can cause weight gain. They can cause dyslipidemia. Surprisingly, olanzapine can cause hyperprolactinemia almost as frequently as risperidone. If you treat with second-generation antipsychotics you must get a *hemoglobin A1c,* a *prolactin level* and a *lipid panel* every few months. You should track *monthly weights.* Don't forget that some of these agents frequently cause akathisia, and less frequently cause all the same side effects as first-generation antipsychotics do. Best: don't use antipsychotics unless an inmate is psychotic.

Reinforcing that, we now have a study that found 80% greater non-injury deaths among people who received "off-label" antipsychotics as children or adolescents—people who were not psychotic.

Bupropion

Bupropion can cause *seizures* when the dose is too large. For this reason the FDA has limited the immediate release (IR) to 150mg. Because the crushed form destroys whatever release control was built into the CR or XL forms, the medication should be limited to 150mg per dose when it is crushed.

Do keep in mind that inmates have been known to crush their bupropion to snort it to get high, exposing them to a risk of seizures.

Lamotrigine

Lamotrigine can cause *Stevens-Johnson syndrome* if it is started abruptly or increased rapidly. SJS is a potentially fatal illness. When an inmate comes in taking lamotrigine, ask her when she last took the med. If more than 4 days have passed she must NOT receive it. Even if it was ordered within the 4-day time frame, if she does not get the med within 4 days, STOP THE MEDICATION.

Because of a variety of factors, it is not safe to start lamotrigine in jails. Don't do it, no matter what an inmate tells you.

Note: Lamotrigine can also induce porphyria accumulation. Be careful with it.

Lithium

The #1 reason for suing psychiatrists is failure to monitor lithium treatment. Get at the very least quarterly blood levels and tests of renal and thyroid functioning. You should monitor kidney functioning yearly. Do not neglect to follow professional guidelines.

Chapter 8
Counseling Inmates

Inmates have a startling ignorance of their internal processes. Often they are afraid of their urges. A surprising number of their complaints can be handled by giving them information rather than chemicals. Perhaps it would not be too much to say that a pinch of insight is worth more than a pound of pills.

And always remember the two rules of therapy: Never Work Harder Than Your Patients Do, and Watch Your Countertransference. For the latter, use your countertransference as a sensor; do not follow it.

ADHD

See Appendix H

Adverse Childhood Experiences

Often inmates come from childhood circumstances, where they were always looking over their shoulders wondering when the next blow would fall and from where. Often people who seemed to be loving relatives would take advantage of the inmate-to-be. When they told their mothers they were being abused, their mothers would slap them across the face and tell them they were liars. The lesson inmates took away from their upbringings is that no one can be trusted. They grow up feeling like no one has their back. Male or female, they develop dysthymia, becoming either borderlines or drug addicts with borderline features.

Women from such backgrounds tend to hook up with men who replicate their abusive fathers or stepfathers. They seem to be looking for some-one who will love them when they were three. They will seek out partners who parent them; but who acts like a parent to an adult partner? A controlling, abusive spouse, that's who! We associate this behavior with borderlines, but this is common to anyone with dysthymia.

Research has shown that borderlines im-prove with time, especially if they find an adult relationship that is stable and loving. So there is hope for people who have been hopeless all their lives. A useful metaphor is the Washington Monu-ment vs the Eiffel Tower. The Washington monu-ment is stone and brick all the way down. It has a solid foundation. Yet the Eiffel tower is taller, and it has nothing but air in its bottom. It comes from nothing, yet there it is. So a person who comes from nothing can make something from his or her life. Such a person can have hope, and should approach therapy with some hope. You will never be able to provide hope with chemicals.

Often persons who go through such ACE's have Complex PTSD.

Adverse Experiences

See also below under "Borderlines."

Blaming God. It is common for an inmate to ask, Why is God letting these bad things happen to me? An answer is that God did not choose to harm you, the perp did.

The first thing to realize is that life is not a video game. When we choose to do good and evil, people are actually helped or harmed by our choices. This is not a video game where we gun down characters that are simply electrons on a screen. You are not a video game character. You are hurt when people beat you or rape you. When a friend or loved one dies, they are gone and you may miss them. Neither you nor they are electrons on a screen. You are all real flesh and blood people.

When harm comes to you, you feel it. When perps choose to do evil and hurt you, then you are hurt. It was the perp who chose to hurt you. Do not blame God or the fates. Blame the perp for choosing to do evil.

Just so, when someone harms you, do not "forgive and forget." That phrase comes from marriage counseling, when one must forget that a spouse has slept with others, or there can be no reconciliation. When someone has harmed you,

you may forgive him, but you should not forget the harm he has done. You should not leave your loved ones where they can be hurt by the perp who hurt you. If a nasty uncle molested you, you should keep your own children out of reach of this monster, keep them safe. Do not forget.

Often persons who go through such ACE's have Complex PTSD.

Anxiety

(See also Appendix G and Chapter 5.)

Most inmates who come to jail feel some worry. Worry is a normal state: inmates worry about what will happen to them; they worry about what will happen to their family, their pets, their belongings; they worry about what their associates will do in their absence. These are legitimate things to worry about. It is normal to worry about these things. In fact, the expression "stayed up all night worrying" reflects how widespread this phenomenon is.

We should not pathologize normal worry by calling it "anxiety." Many people, especially inmates, will describe worry as "anxiety." Yes anxiety shares with worry the fact that are both species of fear. Colloquially, "anxiety" can describe a sense of uneasiness or apprehension. In psychiatry, though, 'anxiety' has been a symptom of a psychiatric illness. As a symptom, anxiety must be an abnormal condition or the marker of an illness. 'Anxiety' is a form of undirected fear or preparation for danger. There is no particular object the sufferer is afraid of or we would use the more accurate term 'fear.'

Some people will shake, either because they are withdrawing from a substance, or because they have a medical condition which causes the shakes, like essential tremor or Parkinson's disease. However, a large number of people will infer that anxiety is causing them to shake.

Some people have difficulty sitting still. They are always restless, on the go, moving their legs in and out, or jiggling them. They can't focus on the task at hand. Rather than call this hyperactivity or ADHD, inmates typically call this "anxiety."

Anxiety is associated with ADHD. It is unclear whether this is an innate symptom or it is learned apprehension that comes from being a hyperactive kid embedded in civilization (always expecting a slap). We will await further research, but note that inmates often give "anxiety" as an excuse for using drugs.

Sometimes inmates are repressing anger. They are afraid they will "lose control." Because of this, they are in conflict. The conflict results in feelings of "anxiety." They feel chest pains, despite being too young to have cardiac pathology. Or the inmate could be lying to you, trying to score some drugs.

On the outside, complaints of anxiety usually bring prescriptions for benzodiazepines. On the inside, if you don't unpack the use of this term, you can be misled as to the actual diagnosis. You may want to prescribe hydroxyzine, diphenhydramine, gabapentin or antipsychotics. But those so-called 'medications' (they are really simply drugs) do not improve the actual conditions; they just cover the symptoms. Consequently, we should not prescribe them.

An inmate may be overly responding to relatively normal circumstances. This is known as an Adjustment Disorder. Jail prescribers do not prescribe anything for Adjustment Disorders. As you may recall, back in the days before the laparoscope was invented, abdominal surgery required large incisions which created a lot of pain. Surgeons then were WW2 vets who knew that long exposure to opiates would produce addicts, so they gave hydroxyzine to people who had surgery. Hydroxyzine is thus a drug (unless you think people who needed surgery were mentally ill). We do not prescribe drugs.

If an inmate truly has anxiety, she must know that her undirected fear puts her in danger. There are dangerous people and situations out there, and she should fear dangerous things. If she does not consciously know that a situation is dangerous, she may still unconsciously know she is in danger. The unconscious communicates this apprehension of danger by signaling fear. She needs to be open to fear signals (sometimes it feels like apprehension; see *The Gift of Fear*, by Gavin deBecker) to avoid dangerous situations. If she feels anxiety—fear of everything—she will blind herself to the signal of real danger—fear of something—that will keep her out of danger. In other words, anxiety is dangerous.

Conquering anxiety is a skill that psychologists can teach. Learning that danger comes from discrete individuals can permit an inmate to descope her fearfulness, to transition from anxiety—fear of everything—to specific fears of dangerous people and dangerous situations. The inmate's overall adjustment will then improve.

Some people will not let go their anxiety. They are familiar with it. In an odd way it is comforting. Except for drugs, they will let nothing treat it. If you do try, understand that; you are not likely to succeed. You might try buspirone here, but don't chase the symptom.

Blaming God

See above under "Adverse Experiences."

Borderlines

Ahh. So frustrating. Everybody hates borderlines, right? Actually the negative countertransference that borderlines engender is provoked on purpose. Perhaps it is done consciously, but more often unconsciously. Borderlines engage in splitting, getting staff to argue with one another. Borderlines engage in splitting, first putting a caregiver on a pedestal then knocking the caregiver off that pedestal. They injure themselves. They can't stand being alone.

If you think of the borderline as having Complex PTSD, some of their actions make sense. Splitting staff, for example, is an exercise of "let's you and him fight"—caregivers are too busy fighting each other to abuse the patient. Engaging in splitting across time, first idolizing then demonizing a caregiver, is trying to test the caregiver, trying to see if the caregiver will go away, like other every significant person in the inmate's life.

Whole books have been written on coping with borderlines. Just remember not to over-respond and especially not to overmedicate the inmate. It is important not to chase symptoms here, because the borderline will always have a new one. Psychotherapy for borderlines is beyond the scope of this book. People with BPD should be referred to others, either for individual or group therapy, like DBT.

A good metaphor for a prescriber is the Eiffel Tower (this time for the prescriber, not the inmate), a tower that stands back from its borders. It is always there. It does not lean over. Just so, the prescriber is always there. The prescriber listens, makes diagnoses and provides appropriate treatment. The prescriber does not pass judgment, does not decide guilt or innocence, does no special favors, never acts like a mother, prescribes no comfort pills. The prescriber may care and let the inmate know that the prescriber does care. But the prescriber gives no special treatment. The prescriber underresponds. When the borderline makes an outrageous statement, the prescriber leaves it alone. The prescriber prescribes appropriate medication, but does not chase symptoms. In the end, the borderline will learn to cope. She always does. Also see above under "Adverse Experiences."

Failure to Appear

Your inmate may be in jail because he has been charged with Failure to Appear. The fact is, this is one charge that is almost guaranteed to get someone put in jail. You may be able get ROR'd on a serious charge but if you don't show up in court—even for a traffic ticket—a warrant will issue for your arrest. The reasoning behind this seems to be that incarceration will assure that you are available to face the charges. I have seen a case where a woman went into a hospital for a heart condition the night before she was due in court. When her lawyer showed up with an explanation, the judge said it didn't matter, and issued a warrant for her arrest. During the next few months while she waited for her turn in court, the inmate was sent from the jail to the hospital several times for her cardiac condition. But 'justice' was served.

Never fail to appear in court. If you know you cannot make the date, call ahead through your lawyer to reschedule. If necessary, show up on a

Gurney (a rolling stretcher) with an IV bag hanging. Never fail to appear when you are due in court, unless you want to come to jail.

Grief

This population seems to have more than their share of losses. Often the losses pile up. They will lose a parent, a job, their spouse, and their home in rapid succession. Friends are killed in MVA's, overdoses and gang violence. Rather than to throw chemicals at the resulting sadness, grief counseling might be in order. Antidepressants might fix an ordinary depression, but even with their depression treated, the losses remain. Sometimes they feel if they sustain one more loss they will kill themselves.

A while ago, grief counseling was part of what clergy did. Now folks turn to mental health folks.

Some things you may wish to ponder: in the normal scheme of things, each generation dies. Great-grandparents, then grandparents, then parents, then you. The next generation will carry on. Your parents don't want to bury you. They would rather have you bury them instead. What you are grieving when your parents die is something selfish: you miss their company, or you missed telling them something important. What saddens you is the timing of the death. The fact of death cannot be escaped.

When friends or sibs die, that is sad. You miss them. But someone has to carry on their memory and it might as well be you. Use your sadness as a monument to the person who passed on. The sadness proves she meant a lot to you.

We do not medicate grief *per se*. In part, this is because doing so only puts off dealing with the loss. In part, this is because a person must learn to deal with losses. Drugs only prevent that. In the society at large, one hopes you the doctor do not use substances when you encounter a loss. Do not prescribe drugs to "help" an inmate deal with loss.

Hyperactivity

See Appendix H

Panic Attacks

Panic attacks are dramatic events often calculated to get caregivers to hurry up and give them a drug. You should resist prescribing anything, even a PRN. The most you should do, is to have a nurse clip on a pulse oximeter to show the inmate she is full of oxygen. The attack will fade. See also Appendix PA.

Parole, Probation, ISP, Drug Court etc.—Alternatives to Incarceration

The term "Probation" will be used in the subsequent discussion to describe all forms of alternatives to incarceration.

Probation is jail with invisible bars. Your primary task while you are on probation, is to please your PO. You start by showing up when he (or she) wants you to. No excuses. If you want to arrange for another date, you must call ahead and get the date formally changed, or go early and hope that will satisfy your PO. If the PO denies permission to change the date, show up when he specifies and show up on time. Even if you have to miss your kid's graduation or a job interview, show up at the PO's office when you are supposed to be there or go to jail. If you have a true conflict, try showing up early and negotiate about the appointment. But if he won't budge, show up.

Other things like not breaking the law and not using drugs (having a "hot urine") are subsidiary. Start with the idea that you will please your PO. He would not want you doing something illegal. If you want to go to a funeral outside your area tell your PO *in advance* and get his permission to go—in writing. Photocopy the permission. Put the original in a safe place. Keep a copy on your person. Do not violate your PO's orders. Do not violate the terms of your probation or parole. Otherwise you will come to jail.

Post-Traumatic Stress Disorder

Our inmates experience all sorts of trauma. You have only to ask about it to get a history. If the person experienced ACE's (Adverse Childhood Experiences) she may not have classic PTSD symptoms. But the trajectory of her life has definitely changed. When this occurs the linkage should be clear to the interviewer.

The person may be able to expunge the ACE's through counseling, or through EMDR. Whatever she chooses, you should encourage her to get that counseling. While you can treat depression with medicines, you cannot expunge the memory of ACE's with pills. Have some humility, doc.

See also Appendix PT.

Quiet Panic Attacks

Some borderlines complain of "panic attacks" when they have nothing of the sort. They may sit quietly next to your desk complaining of the "panic" that they feel. This is one of the reasons you should unpack the term each and every time you come to it. The inmate may not mean the same thing you do when she uses the word.

Smoking

In AA and NA they stress the importance of changing People, Places and Things to break free of an addiction. They say nothing of changing Faces, Places and Things, despite the attraction of saying something that rhymes. Why not?

If all you change is the specific people you hang out with, you have changed the particular faces without changing the *kind* of people you hang out with. They will still be the same kind of users you used to know. Among smokers, everybody drinks. If you ask a group of nonsmokers if nonalcoholic punch is OK, they will drink it. If you ask a bunch of smokers, they will hoot you out of the place; they want their alcohol.

Smoking is one of the last legal discriminations. Smokers make up 20% of the population. Typically they are shunned by the other 80%. Few nonsmokers will abide smoking. A few nonsmokers may mix with smokers, but not many, and not for long. When a smoker looks out at the world, all he sees is other smokers; the 80% who don't smoke make themselves scarce. They avoid smokers.

Nonsmokers can smell smokers. If you even share an elevator with someone who has come in from outside on her smoke break, when you get back to your own office your nonsmoking colleagues will remark on how you smell like smoke. Imagine if you reek of cigarettes that you yourself have smoked.

So the power of a comment like "You will find most of your drinkers and drug-users among the smokers" hits home. That truthful comment says that drinkers and drug-users are mostly concentrated among that 20%.

We will also note that a cigarette habit is expensive: a pack-a-day habit costs $200 a month. It gets more expensive as you smoke more.

Want to quit using drugs or alcohol? Save some money? Then quit smoking, and start hanging around nonsmokers.

Stress

Everybody experiences stress. It could come with the demands of daily life. It could come from life in the jail. Maybe someone has died. Maybe the inmate is worrying about their family and how they are doing without the inmate being there to help. Another word for this is worry.

We do not medicate stress. Stress is something you cope with, metabolize. We do not medicate worry. These things are part of normal life and we learn to cope with normal life.

If someone develops a depression while they are coping with life's stressors, we can treat that. With SSRI's. We do not treat the depression that results from stress with antipsychotics, benzodiazepines, diphenhydramine, hydroxyzine, mirtazapine, TCA's or trazodone. Instead, we treat with SSRI's or with SNRI's like venlafaxine or duloxetine. If an inmate is looking for a comfort pill, she should look elsewhere.

Substances

If you are doing substances, you can't be a good parent. You are focused on getting your drugs, not taking care of your children. You are drug-centered or alcohol-centered, not kid-centered. If you want to take care of your kids, ditch the drugs or alcohol. See also Chapter 6.

Suicidal Ideation

See Appendix S.

Tremor

A lot of people shake. A lot of inmates believe that if they are shaking, they must be anxious. Causes for tremulousness are numerous, including (but not limited to) withdrawal effects, essential tremor, side effects of a medication (including lithium, T4 and various anticonvulsants), toxicity from poisons or other chemicals, adrenaline, thyroid hormone, Parkinson's disease and other medical causes. Just because someone has a tremor does not mean she is feeling anxious.

Unhappiness

Most people who come to jail are unhappy. They say they are "depressed" and "anxious," saying they will become "violent" with their peers. All of this is more or less normal on entering a place of incarceration. Jails are not meant to be nice places, and one's freedom of action has been formally taken away. If a person was not engaged in psychiatric treatment before coming to jail, or if a person was not having psychiatric symptoms before coming to jail, then the inmate may simply be responding to incarceration, withdrawing from substances, or both. Such a person might benefit from a mental health counselor coming around to visit. Or such an inmate might benefit from group therapy.

Violence and the Potential for Violence

We must all reckon with our "inner chimp." Nature videos are so very instructive. They show the actions of animals who share 96% of our genome. The male chimpanzee is violent. Individually and in gangs male chimpanzees routinely maim and kill smaller monkeys and each other. They are strong enough that they can take a smaller monkey and literally rip him limb from limb. Systematic studies back up these casual observations.

So as human beings we all do battle with our "inner chimp," our violent urges; and we are surprisingly successful at it. We live together in large communities, aggregates of individuals large enough to make any chimp "go ape." Despite that, we are usually more or less civil to each other.

Some inmates may fear that they will "lose it" and "black out," visiting violence on others. Yet for the most part their peers are as big and strong as they are, often bigger and stronger. Not to mention group vengeance. So there are social curbs on an inmate's behavior.

That assumes that an inmate is honestly re-flecting his inner urges. However, inmates often threaten violence in order to convince the doctor to prescribe drugs. These inmates have a sense that we all have inner urges to violence, so their threats sound realistic. But they are not really interested in assistance in controlling their urges. They want drugs.

The approach here is not to prescribe drugs. Instead acknowledge the urge to violence but as a normal feeling. Point to chimpanzees as an example of wild behavior and note that all of us live in a civilization full of people with violent emotions inside. We all control ourselves.

The task of adolescence is to channel that inner rage into something constructive. Not all of us manage that; some plunge into drugs, for example. But almost all of us curtail those violent impulses, especially when there are external constraints. Jail is the quintessence of external constraints on one's behavior. So, for the most part, inmates do not need meds to help with control themselves, much less drugs. In the end, you can always put an inmate on house-alone status to protect others.

Worry

See Stress. See also Anxiety and Quiet Panic Attacks.

Your Way

I will repeat the story about the poster I found on the wall when I first came to work in a jail:

This is not Burger King, and you can't have it your way. Try to remember that having it your way got you here.

It is surprising how many inmates think they can get their way by acting out. After all, in prior situations they always got their way.

Jails have been literally dealing for centuries with inmates who are trying to get their way by bullying or intimidating others. They are bound to be disappointed. Although you can point this out to an inmate, the inmate is likely to be "hard-headed" about this. In the 19th century people

who did not seem to be able to learn from experience were called "moral idiots." That tells us that
some problems do not fade away.

Chapter 9
Your Note

Your note falls into one of two types: the initial contact and the progress note.

Initial Note:

Demographics Age, marital status, race, date of commitment, and whether on a withdrawal protocol. E.g.—"42yo MBM DOC 7/1/19 on Librium w/d prot for etoh."

The age, marital status and whether or not the inmate has children will later figure into the inmate's suicidality.

If you see the inmate who was on a withdrawal protocol within a month of his coming to jail, you know he is still in the detox phase of his coming off his drugs or alcohol (or both). If such a person was in active psychiatric treatment before coming to jail, you can treat what he was in treatment for—if it was a legitimate psychiatric disorder. Otherwise you may be listening to detox complaints, complaints from a brain that is screaming for its missing substances. In such a case, it may be wise to wait a while longer. and to see the inmate until after the detox phase has passed. Sometimes when a person goes through detox, he emerges in good spirits no longer in need of psychiatric services—or psychiatric meds.

When a person comes in who was committed to jail some months before but only now is showing up with complaints of depression, that inmate may have been worn down by the circumstances of incarceration. That inmate may actually be depressed. That is the inmate where you expect to find something to treat.

Reason for Referral/Chief Complaint What is the inmate asking for? I usually put down quotations here. Like "I need something to sleep" (usually an indicator of ADHD) or "I take medicine on the street for my bipolar." Rarely someone will come in saying he takes paroxetine on the street, and wants to avoid a discontinuation syndrome. Normally, it is someone looking for drugs.

Sometimes you must pry the chief complaint out of an inmate. You can ask "What can I do for you?" or "Why are you here to see me?" or "What problems do you have that you need to see a psychiatrist?" I'm sure you can think of other ways of framing this.

History This is usually blown off as "social history." But that's not what this is. A social history is all about whether the inmate is married or living with another and how many kids are involved and how many children the child welfare services have taken away. No, this is about the inmate's early years. See Chapter 4 for details.

Substances You are not interested in casual use. You are interested in daily or regular use. You want to know what substances the inmate is or has been dependent on. You might ask the age someone started his/her marijuana, alcohol or drugs. This will give you an approximate guide to the person's emotional age.

Past Medical History (PMH) You need to write NKDA to show that you have asked this.

Be sure to cover any medical problems like diabetes, hepatitis (A,B,C), hypertension, seizure disorders, sickle cell, sleep apnea, etc.

History of the Present Illness (HPI) (Also: Psychiatric History) Cover the history of suicide attempts, suicide gestures, self-injurious behavior (SIB) and psychiatric admissions, such as "2 suic atts from 16yo to 4 mo ago. 3 psych adms for SI and SIB from 16yo to last week. Distressed (or not) when alone."

You are looking to learn if this inmate is liable to attempt suicide, make a suicide gesture or injure herself. You are looking for admissions for mania or psychosis. Also, any history of self-injury goes here. Finally, you are looking for a history of actual (not threatened) injury to others.

After getting the basic "psychiatric demo-graphics" you can proceed to cover past and current psychiatric treatment history. If an inmate has suffered traumas as an adult, cover it here. Basically you are explaining how an adult's psychiatric illness developed. This may be sketchy, however, as most of an inmate's sorrows may stem from troubles suffered in childhood or adolescence.

Mental Status Examination (MSE) A MSE is like the physical examination. Like the PE it cannot be omitted from a psychiatric evaluation. If you write down a MSE every time you see an inmate you will have reference points; you will have the inmate's state documented each time you have seen him. More: if an inmate is leaving clues that his history is feigned, you can record it here.

Impression (Imp) Here is where you can get away with "doing well." If the inmate is not doing well you can document that. Sometimes you will have to explain that despite objective observations of normalcy, an inmate is not doing well. Or even though he is expressing a lot of pathology, you think it is all fake. Ideally, of course, you will record the clues as you see them, but sometimes the malingering comes to you, when you try to put the clinical picture together. You have to record that somewhere, so you might as well do it here.

If the condition is complicated, the Impression section is where to record your formulation. You can describe how the pieces fit together.

Diagnosis (Dx) Traditionally, the diagnosis at the top shows the condition that is being addressed by whatever specialist is seeing the patient. You certainly could do that. However, psychiatry is a specialty that addresses multiple diagnoses. Typically, we are dealing with the entire burden of trials and tribulations that have accumulated over the years to trouble a patient. Think that troubles are not cumulative? Try sitting with an 85-year-old woman, crying about molestations that happened to her when she was five years old. Eighty years might have passed, but she was still suffering. For that reason, a list of the current diagnoses in chronological order of age of onset makes sense.

As this is written, we have passed out of DSM-IV and moved on to DSM-5. That means No More Axes. That old impediment to a chronological list of troubles has been removed. Further, we have moved from ICD-9 to ICD-10 and are getting ready for ICD-11. This all will affect how you record your diagnoses.

An example:

F88	ND-PAE [a prenatal diagnosis]
F90	ADHD [an early onset diagnosis]
F43.12	complex PTSD [or F34.1 Dysthymia, both early childhood diagnoses]
F60.3	BPD [arguably a form of Complex PTSD]
F19.2	PSD [polysubstance dependence; usually starts in adolescence]
F32.9	Depression NOS [the inmate may be in rehab from her drugs]

The last may be the only condition she has that is addressable in jail with medications, though the inmate's having ADHD may affect your choice of medication.

You may object that the diagnosis of personality disorders has changed with DSM-5. There are dimensions now. Well, the eggheads that came up with that should stick to doing research. Busy clinicians will have no time for it. We will continue to diagnose personalities, when they depart from normal, as distinct syndromes. As if to acknowledge that, DSM-5 continues to provide us with those diagnoses.

Plan Be sure to write down what your plan is. Write down the meds, the dosages, and what they are for. If you anticipate various contingencies, write them down so that if a colleague must cover for you, she will see what you are doing, and can follow your plan.

In summary:

Demographics
RFR/CC - Reason for Referral/Chief Complaint
Hx - History
Subst - Substances
PMH - Past Medical History
HPI - History of the Present Illness
MSE - Mental Status Examination
Imp - Impression
Dx - Diagnosis
Plan

Re-Intake Note:

This is where your preparation can pay big dividends. You have already gathered 90% of what you need to know. In essence, you can refer to your past note and remark on what has occurred for the inmate since he left the jail the last time. Then you write down your MSE, formulated your diagnoses and make your plans. Then you are done.

Demographics, including a reference to past notes on IM
RFR/CC - Reason for Referral/Chief Complaint
Updates, if any
MSE - Mental Status Examination
Imp - Impression
Dx - Updated Diagnosis
Plan

Progress Note:

Some people believe that you should use the SOAP format for progress notes. When you consider that the SOAP note is supposed to be part of a pervasive problem-oriented medical record system and that this system was conceived without psychiatric input, you can begin to see how woefully inappropriate this system is for psychiatric progress notes.

Timing The NCCHC requires that IM's be seen every three months at a minimum. Of course, if the inmate needs to be seen before that, he should be seen when clinically indicated. Otherwise see inmates every two months to assure inmates will be seen before the three-month clock is up. That way, if you or the mental health team make a mistake, or the inmate is not available, you can do a follow-up appointment before the three months have passed. Don't write the requirement down, or you will be held to the shorter period.

Current Treatment You should record the current medications and doses the inmate is supposed to be taking, if any. If you have access to the MAR's, you can comment on the inmate's compliance. If you don't, you will have to ask the inmate whether he is taking his meds.

Current Status/Progress How is she doing? Has her depression subsided? Have the voices faded? Comment on whether the inmate is having any trouble with her medications. Based on the issues you identified in your intake note and previous progress notes, how has the inmate progressed on her various problems? This should be about your most straightforward section.

Medical Status/Progress You should ask the inmate how he has been doing medically. You can track issues that have been problems for the inmate. In particular, if the inmate is taking one of the second-generation antipsychotic meds, you must track the inmate's weight, his hemoglobin A1c and his lipids. For risperidone or olanzapine, get a prolactin level. If the patient is taking lithium, carbamazepine or divalproex, you will want to get levels.

MSE Your MSE can be a little shortened here if you handwrite your notes. If you have established that an inmate has no trouble with psychosis, you can replace the sections on flow of thought (FOT), responding to internal stimuli (RIS; hallucinations) and presence of delusions expressed or elicited with the statement "Nonpsychotic." You could also skip the memory and intellect statements if you are pressed for time. However the Appearance section of your mental status should include a statement on the presence or absence of signs and symptoms of EPS or tardive dyskinesia (TD) if your inmate is taking antipsychotic medications, especially first generation.

Imp (Impression) If the inmate is doing well or struggling, comment here. The statement may be brief or long, but the better you explain your thinking the easier it will be for a colleague or you to later see what you were thinking at the time of the note.

Dx If you handwrite your notes, you can update your **diagnosis** every several times you see inmates. If you are using an EHR you can copy the diagnosis and paste it into your current note.

Plan This is the same as for the initial note: Write down the meds, the dosages, and what they are for. If you anticipate various contingencies, write them down so that if a colleague must cover for you she will see what you are doing and can follow your plan.

Tx	Current treatment
Prog	Current Status/Progress
PMH	Medical Status/Progress
MSE	Mental Status Examination
Imp	Impression
Dx	(updated if necessary)
Plan	Plan, in detail if needed

Electronic Healthcare Record (EHR)

See also Appendix E.

When you are using one of these, you can automate a number of tasks. Some EHR's allow a text replacement functionality. This allows you to speed up your input phenomenally.

If you have a **browser-based EHR**, you should keep sections of text in separate files so you can copy and paste whole blocks of text. Why? Because **an errant keystroke can lose you everything with no hope of recovery.**

Ideally the blocks of text have lots of options so you can prune them to fit the inmate. Be wary when pasting text, however. You will want to edit what you have just pasted and prune out the inappropriate words.

You can also use an Autotext or autocorrect function. It beats typing them out but you must be ready with the delete key. An example: You type "fu." With the text replacement function you get "IM seen for routine follow-up. Current medication order:" then you invoke the special paste function where you insert the current med orders into your note.

This is followed by "ls" (small case "LS") which transforms into "Last seen:" where you enter the date. In the prior note, you have the Impression followed by the Plan. These can be copied as a block and pasted into your current progress note. You can then type out the inmate's progress, his response to meds, etc. You next discuss any medical issues that have arisen. You may have access to laboratory data. You should enter it here either by pasting or typing. Finally, you enter your MSE. Your MSE will probably contain many alternates, which you delete to fit this particular inmate.

When you are done, you can invoke "Impression:" and type out what you think about the inmate's progress. At the end, you have a plan; meds prescribed, consultations made, labs ordered. You may have some post-release recommendations. In any case, make your note intelligible to you and helpful to you. And recall that diligent nurses will be reading your notes for guidance. Make your note intelligible and helpful for them, too.

Try to write your note with enough detail that another professional can read it and see why you made your diagnoses. Ideally, the note has enough detail that others can make their own diagnoses from your notes.

Printed History and MSE

In a handwritten form, you may wish to reduce your writing. Below are specimens. Remember, these forms merely eliminate repetitive writing. They do not replace telling your inmate's story.

These specimens are reproduced in 12-point fonts. In the original form, they are in 9-point text.

You will note that the questions are framed in a Yes/No, Choice/No or Choice/Denies format. The presence of '/N' or '/Denies' shows that you asked the question. Leaving it uncircled, implies that you did not ask the question.

'D/A' means 'drug addict /alcoholic.'

When someone answers the question in a non-standard way, explain it in detail in your note. For example, if someone indicates she was molested, you write down who molested her at what ages, and what someone did when they were told at the time. If someone is drowsy, circle the N and in your note write that the inmate was drowsy.

"Special ed" includes behavior classes, resource rooms, etc.

Raised in US / NJ / Other   by Parents / Mother / GM / Other

Mother D/A / N Father D/A / N   Step-Father D/A /N/Unk

Mother Drank/Used While Preg Y / N / Don't know

As Child: Verbal Abuse Y / N Beaten Y / N   Molested Y / N

Trouble: sitting still Y / N Paying Attn Y / N   Impulsive Y / N

Trouble Getting to sleep at night Y / N   In special ed Y / N

Ritalin / Adderall / Other ADD med Proposed / Unk / N

Socialized When Young Y / N   Distressed When Alone Y / N

Suicide Attempt/Gesture Y / N   h/o Self-Injury Y / N

Psychiatric Admission Y / N   Detox/Rehab Adm Y / N

Alert/ N Bouncing/Wiggling Leg/Foot/ N   Normoactive Y / N

Euthymic/Neutral/Low/Sad/Worried/Anxious/Irritated/Angry

Approp. Affect Y / N   Smiles & Laughs Spont & Approp. Y / N

FOT WNL Y / N RIS / N Delusions Y/ N   Wants to live Y / N

HI / Denies Current Voices Y/ Denies   Suicidal Id Y/ Denies

Ox3 / N Mem Intact Y / N Intel Fx WNL Y / N   I&J Fair / N

Chapter 10
Special Circumstances

Assault

Alas, occasionally an inmate will assault a clinician. Such an occurrence is thankfully rare. Most likely the assault will come from a psychotic inmate. Such an inmate may, for example, think he can escape by running from his cell. If you are standing at the entrance of the cell between him and what he supposes is freedom he may toss you and make a run for it. The fact that he has only escaped to the larger jail will now dawn on him. One solution for this is to have a CO between you and the inmate.

Even better, you can interview a psychotic inmate through the lunch hole—the slot through which a food tray enters and leaves a cell. Or an inmate will be brought to you in handcuffs or other shackles. Do not agitate to have the cuffs removed.

If an inmate sits and talks to you then spits on you—that is an assault. In many jurisdictions it is an assault with a deadly weapon (spittle is considered a deadly weapon because it can transmit deadly diseases).

You must not "forgive" an inmate for assaulting you. This is a matter of safety. The inmate must know that assaulting any staff will get him street charges 100% of the time. If he assaults you, he assumes he can assault me, and his buddies think they can assault medical staff. Whatever charges he would get if he assaulted a CO is the least charge he should get for assaulting non-CO staff.

Custody vs Clinical

Sometimes CO's do not talk to inmates. Sometimes they just bring the inmate to Mental Health. The inmate then complains of issues that involve Custody, not Mental Health. In such cases, direct the inmate to refer all her inquiries to Custody, not Mental Health. Do not get in the middle of it. Do not act as a go-between. Do not "translate" the inmate to the correctional authorities; do not "explain" routine institutional practices to the inmate. This is triangulation. Do not involve yourself in it. The most you can do is suggest IA.

Hole, The

The inmate may be in "The Hole." This is otherwise known as "lock-up." This is a form of confinement, usually solo, initiated by CO's for problematic inmates. Strictly speaking, it is not a punishment.

Interview Circumstances

An inmate may object to being interviewed in a "public" space. He may object to giving his history with a CO standing over him maintaining watch. Perhaps an inmate talks so softly he cannot be heard. Perhaps an inmate objects to inquiries about his early life, complaining that it is not relevant—to his purpose of getting drugs.

Regardless of circumstances, the inmate is coming to you for meds. Unless the inmate adapts to the circumstances, he can go away without meds. Let the inmate talk louder so he can be heard. If a soft-spoken inmate (speaking softly is a tactic) suddenly gets loud, then a CO moves from the periphery to up-close and the inmate loses what privacy he had. Now he says nothing. In such a circumstance, he remains on one-to-one suicide watch and gets no meds. Maybe he is allowed no blanket or clothing, apart from his suicide gown. Perhaps he was truly suicidal. Perhaps he was not suicidal but will do some act of self-injury or suicide gesture if released. In any case, he is protected if you leave him on one-to-one. He is motivated to quit his manipulative behavior in favor of the promise of pills. But no amount of chemicals will stop a determined inmate. Best to let him put on his show, until he gets tired of play-acting.

Juveniles

Juveniles are not different from adults. They are just earlier along in the process of whatever makes them dysfunctional. Some of them are criminals in training, learning their eventual craft. It is interesting to see them in the process of making their moral choices, learning how to lie, cheat and steal. If you think you can stop them, you are sadly mistaken. Intervening by treating a criminal's ADHD, while it sounds good in theory, does not appear to work on the inmates who come to jail.

There are others who have been badly hurt. It is possible that you may get them aimed at the therapy they need. But don't let the little jewels gain anything by lying to you (one young hoodlum wanted me to talk to his deceased mother as he left the interview room, patting the air as if patting the shoulder of a pookah). Observe the principals of good psychiatric practice. Do not enable anyone. First of all, do no harm.

Lock-Up

See discussion under "Hole, The."

Pregnancy

Most of us are not certified addiction medicine specialists, so if a pregnant woman comes in on methadone, we must leave her on the same dose of methadone. Notice how mother-centered this is: the resulting child will be born addicted to an opiate and will need to go through some sort of withdrawal. This seems to be a nasty trick to play on a newborn, but there it is.

By extension, there is a move afoot to continue benzodiazepines if a pregnant female is taking alprazolam or something similar. Benzodiazepines are all contraindicated in pregnancy. Your general medical specialist should convert the woman to clonazepam and taper her down—if the benzodiazepine was prescribed. To give a pregnant woman benzodiazepines on her say-so to compensate for non-prescribed benzodiazepines she alleges she was taking, invites women to lie about their benzodiazepine intake.

Further, there is one legitimate psychiatric medication you can safely prescribe to a pregnant inmate. Other meds are soporific and not prescribed. Buspirone alone seems to have both a psychiatric indication and is category B, or OK to use in pregnancy.

You are safest to prescribe nothing but psychotherapy to a woman in jail who is pregnant.

Preparation

Sometimes your associates see an inmate before you do, preparing extensive reports and notes. In some circumstances, CO's will bring an inmate to you. If you take too much time, you will be burning CO time. These situations can collide to give you no time to read in advance. Perhaps the information provided to you, does not prepare you for the amount of pre-interview reading you must do to see an inmate. Take the time to pre-read the information. You may keep the CO's waiting, but that is a matter of scheduling and pre-interview notification. You can't be everywhere and do everything.

Psych Clearance

You will be asked to "clear" an inmate for general population. The topic will be discussed under "Suicide Watch" and Appendix S.

Restraint

Most confinement facilities will have one or more restraint chairs for inmates. These are superior to "four-point" restraints in a number of respects. Properly done, a person can be restrained in a chair with relatively loose straps. How? By holding both sides of a person's elbow, for example, the person cannot get out. In a traditional four-point restraint, a person could ooze out of a restraint by sliding his hands through wrist restraints that were not tight enough. Getting restraints "tight enough" without stopping circulation was difficult. In a restraint chair, wrist restraints can be much looser and still hold the inmate in.

Another reason a restraint chair is superior to a supine four-point restraint, is that the latter is too similar to a rape position. The restraint chair avoids that. Finally, a restraint chair allows for elimination in place without having to allow release from the chair to allow an inmate to go to the bathroom.

An inmate may be restrained because he was injuring himself, banging his head on the wall. When housing an inmate alone in a cell is not enough to keep him safe, CO's will resort to the restraint chair. But CO's don't want to order the restraint chair themselves. They want you to do it. Don't.

Afterword:
How to be a Jailhouse Shrink

At the end of Chapter 3, we saw the document that started this book. How did we do? On the next several pages, we have an updated set of treatment guidelines. Doubtless, in the future it will be updated yet again.

Guidelines for Jail Psychiatry, 2019

Remember Loeb's Laws:

- First of all, do no harm.
- If what you're doing works, keep doing it.
- If what you're doing doesn't work, stop doing it.
- Never make the treatment worse than the disease.

Have some humility doc: you can't treat everything with pills.

We do not treat insomnia.

We do not treat anxiety.

Psychiatrists do not treat withdrawal in jails. Further, if an inmate is having problems, it may involve intoxication or detox, which is the period that follows withdrawal.

Psychiatrists do not treat seizures or pain or other medical conditions.

We never ever prescribe benzodiazepines for any reason whatsoever.

We do not treat ADD/ADHD unless the CO's complain about the inmate's behavior.

We never ever prescribe stimulants.

Always remember that inmates lie, especially to get drugs. They are better liars than you are a lie detector.

Always be open to reports from nurses and CO's who observe an inmate when you are not present.

For depression, use an SSRI first, then try an SNRI. In no case prescribe a desirable "comfort pill." Meds are normally QAM.

While you already know that we do not order benzodiazepines (alcohol in a pill), we also do not order hydroxyzine. It used to be that we ordered hydroxyzine after a major surgery. People who get major surgery are not mentally ill, so hydroxyzine is a drug. We don't prescribe drugs.

We only prescribe medications on-label in a jail, so we do not order gabapentin and topiramate. Those meds have not earned any psychiatric indications, so psychiatrists do not prescribe them in a jail.

We only order antipsychotics in a jail for psychosis. We never order these medicines for anxiety, ADHD symptoms or sleep.

Because antipsychotics can and do cause diabetes, dyslipidemia (including high cholesterol) and obesity, do labs every few months, and keep track of monthly weights. BTW—olanzapine is #2 behind risperidone in causing hyperprolactin-emia, or "man boobs." Quetiapine is famous among inmates because it is like heroin, so we do not prescribe it at all. The only antipsychotics on our formulary are haloperidol, risperidone and olanzapine. Aripiprazole may join them soon.

We only prescribe diphenhydramine when it accompanies an antipsychotic. Alone, it can be a sleeping pill, which we do not prescribe. If I had my way, we would not prescribe it at all, but benztropine has gotten too expensive to use on a regular basis.

Mirtazapine is an excellent antidepressant at 30mg to 45mg per day. Less than that, it is not an effective antidepressant—just a sleeping pill. We do not order mirtazapine at all, because it is diverted and sold or bartered in the jail. If an inmate has been taking it, find an alternate.

Bupropion is an excellent antidepressant, but it is crushed and snorted by inmates like speed. Thus, as a drug of abuse, it is not ordered. Recall that bupropion was withdrawn when it first came out, because it caused seizures. It came back with a cap of 150mg per dose and even now faces an SR cap of 200mg. A higher dose than 200mg must be the XL form.

In place of bupropion, try venlafaxine XL. Straight venlafaxine is a not as effective on the average and requires that our nurses give it multiple times a day. Venlafaxine XL is given once a day. It is approved for depression, anxiety, social phobia ("paranoia" according to inmates) and may help with ADHD. The only trouble with venlafaxine is dose-finding. I start with XL 37.5mg QAM for 2 weeks then automatically increase the dose to 75mg QAM. This gives the inmate time to tell his/her nurse that the current dose is just fine. The next steps are 150mg QAM and 300mg QAM.

Other antidepressants that we use: fluoxetine, sertraline, paroxetine and citalopram. Usually the first med we try is citalopram, which has an FDA-mandated cap of 40mg QD. We do not use escitalopram, because it is just a form of citalopram. If you must use it, a non-formulary application for it will probably get approved. For anxiety not responsive to antidepressants, we can prescribe buspirone.

Inmates use words differently from how you were trained (see Appendix G). "Anxiety," for example, often means the inmate cannot sit still, cannot pay attention and cannot sleep at night. Of course these are symptoms of ADHD, which has about a 90% prevalence in a psychiatric jail population (using identical screening tools I got about a 5% prevalence of ADHD in a general hospital). "Antisocial" is used to describe social withdrawal. "Paranoid" often means social phobia. "Night terrors" usually means nightmares, often associated with traumatic events. So always find out what an inmate means when he/she uses a technical term. When they say "depressed," for example, they usually mean they are merely unhappy and they consider it a normal response to an adverse circumstance (ICD-10 has a code for that: Z65.1 Incarceration).

TCA's must never be used in a jail population. Someone will be stupid enough to take an overdose while trying to get high. We don't need that kind of death, so no TCA's.

If someone is taking a TCA or an SNRI and claim they have "bipolar disorder" you know the inmate does not have real bipolar disorder: anything that depends on stimulating the adrenergic system—like TCA's, duloxetine, mirtazapine or venlafaxine—will destabilize a true bipolar disorder. Think dysthymia or BPD instead.

As psychiatrists in a jail, we do not prescribe nonpsychiatric meds. This includes blood pressure meds like clonidine and prazosin. If an inmate wants one of those, he/she must see our medical specialist.

The VA has been looking for a chemical treatment for PTSD for 50 years. They have not found one yet (they have even tried prazosin and gotten equivocal results). So don't prescribe antipsychotics for PTSD. Stick with an antidepressant.

Be sure to write down all the diagnoses you find, and write down your plan. Also, if you have recommendations like EMDR for PTSD, or seeing a family doctor to treat ADHD, write those down, too. Then tell the inmate she/he can get a copy of your report sent to her/his outpatient provider if the inmate signs a release of information.

BTW—I call benzodiazepines "alcohol in a pill" for good reasons: you will do stupid stuff you would not do without it (disinhibition; inmates call it the "felony pill"), you won't remember what you did (impaired memory; the "amnesia pill"), they impair sleep architecture and the withdrawal syndrome is exactly like alcohol, with withdrawal seizures, visual hallucinations, delirium tremens, etc. Benzodiazepines have no place in psychiatry. It's like giving someone a drink when she/he is upset.

Psychiatric meds used here:

Citalopram	Buspirone
Duloxetine	Haloperidol
Fluoxetine	Olanzapine
Paroxetine	Risperidone
Sertraline	Amantadine
Venlafaxine XR	Benztropine
Carbamazepine	Diphenhydramine
Divalproex	Trihexyphenidyl
Oxcarbazepine	Lithium

Appendix AA
Acronyms and
Abbreviations

An acronym is a word made from the initials of a term. An abbreviation is the shortening of a word. The acronyms and abbreviations below are not always strictly medical, but you will find them in charts, so they are decoded here. Be aware that the identical acronyms or abbreviations may have different meanings in different contexts.

↑	Increase, Increased
↓	Decrease, Decreased
2°	Secondary to; due to
A	When used as part of a SOAP note: Assessment
A1c	Hemoglobin A1c, a marker for diabetes
AA	Alcoholics Anonymous
AC	Latin for Before Meals
ACOA	(or ACA) Adult Child Of Alcoholic. The concept outlines some of the characteristics of a person who was raised by an alcoholic, especially; or more generally, raised by any substance abuser.
ACE	Adverse Childhood Experience(s). In context, Angiotensin Converting Enzyme
ACT	Assertive Community Treatment. See also PACT.
A/D	Alcoholic/Drug-addicted. Usually used in

the negative, as in "Raised by parents (who were) not A/D."

AD   Active Duty. The phase of military service that follows training.

ADD   Attention Deficit Disorder (F90.0)

ADH   Anti-Diuretic Hormone

ADHD   Attention Deficit Hyperactivity Disorder

ADL   Activities of Daily Living

adj   Adjusted, adjustment

AH   Auditory Hallucinations

AIT   Advanced Individual Training. A course for Army recruits to train for a military specially; follows basic training (BCT), precedes active duty (AD). Doesn't involve the other services.

AMPD   Alternative Model of Personality Disorders. A model that that shows some promise. The ICD-11 concept of personality disorders apparently tracks this.

alt   Alternative, as in "alternative school"

alter   Alternate personality. Seen in DID.

ANC   Absolute Neutrophil Count. Used in clozapine therapy.

anx   Anxiety, anxious. Beware when patients tell you they are "anxious;" they may mean ADHD symptoms, or that they are scared. See Appendix G and Chapter 5.

APN   Advanced Practice Nurse (e.g.—Nurse Practitioner)

APS   Adult Protective Services. A branch of government in some states, for protecting older adults who may be physically, financially or psychologically abused by someone.

ARBD Alcohol Related Birth Defects

ARND Alcohol-Related Neurodevelopmental Disorder

ASA Acetyl-Salicylic Acid

ASD Autism Spectrum Disorder

assoc Associated, association

ASPD Also ASP. Antisocial Personality Disorder. Because drug addicts often engage in antisocial acts to support their habits, and because we do not have time to collect the accurate history of an inmate's childhood that would support a diagnosis of ASPD, we really cannot diagnose this with any accuracy. Further, people with paranoid schizophrenia can become markedly antisocial when they develop their illness. Obviously, they develop their antisocial tendencies late, so a diagnosis of ASPD cannot be made. For a jail population, this is most often a useless diagnosis. If antisocial tendencies need to be noted, the term "with antisocial features" can be appended to a diagnosis.

ATM At The Moment. Borrowed from texting. In non-medical contexts it may mean Automatic Teller Machine.

atty Attorney

aud Auditory. In context, audible

AVH Auditory and Visual Hallucinations

B, (B) Brother. In typing, an uppercase B; in handwriting. a B with a circle around it.

BAC   Blood Alcohol Content

BAD   A really "bad" acronym for Bipolar Affect-ive Disorder. Use BD instead.

BAL   Blood Alcohol Level

BBB   Blood-Brain Barrier. In this context, it is not the Better Business Bureau.

BCT   Basic Combat Training. The first stage of an Army recruit's training. Today nine weeks, the course length has varied. It precedes AIT. Does not apply to the other services. In the Navy or the Marines the initial training is "Boot Camp."

BD   Bipolar Disorder. Preferred form.

BDD   Body Dysmorphic Disorder

BDS   An acronym sometimes used instead of BID, especially abroad. It stands for the Latin Bis Die Sumendum or 'take twice a day.' You might run into it.

behav Behavior, Behavioral, etc. Preferred abbrev. for these words. Do not use 'Bx.'

benzo Benzodiazepine. Deprecated. Use BZD.

BID   international medical abbreviation: Bis In Die. Latin for 'twice a day.' Some facilities mean a specific timing when this is written, but this really only means 'twice a day' and nothing more.

BIF   Borderline Intellectual Functioning—IQ nominally 70-85. ICD-10 R41.83.

bilat Bilateral

BIPAP Bilevel Positive Airway Pressure—a proprietary form of CPAP.

BLM   Buccal-Lingual Movements. Common element of TD (Tardive Dyskinesia)

BMP   Basic Metabolic Profile. A Medicare-approved lab test for electrolytes. They specified the abbreviation as well. Similar to SMA-6.

BPD   Borderline Personality Disorder. In context, it may mean Bags Per Day.

BSO   Bilateral Salpingo-Oophorectomy

BTA   Botulinum Toxin A

BTW   From online use. It means 'by the way.'

bx   Do not use this. Used by mental health workers who have not been medically trained to mean 'behav,' but in medical usage, bx has long been the abbreviation for 'biopsy.' Your using it for any other purpose would be confusing.

BZD   Benzodiazepine(s)

BZO   Benzodiazepine. Deprecated. Use BZD instead.

c   [handwritten abbrev: small c with a line over it] International medical abbreviation for 'with,' from Latin 'cum.' For typewritten abbrev, use 'w/.'

ca   Cancer. Outside of medicine, it is short for 'circa,' or Canada.

CABG   Coronary Artery Bypass Graft. A CABG is *not* "open heart surgery:" the heart is not opened.

CBC   Complete Blood Count

CBD   Cannabidiol, a component of MJ

CBT   Cognitive Behavior Therapy. A manualized form of structured psychotherapy.

CBZ   Carbamazepine

CD   Conduct Disorder, a necessary precursor to ASPD. Outside medicine, it has many meanings.

CFS   Child and Family Services. An arm of a state government. In other states, similar offices are CPS, CYS, DYFS, etc.

CFA   Confirmatory Factor Analysis. A term used in clinical research

CHF   Congestive Heart Failure

CJ   County Jail

CM   Case Manager. For SPMI patients who do not need intense services. A case manager may help a patient get to appointments, show up at court, fill out applications for Disability status, get medications, etc. A more intense service would be an ICM: Intensive Case Manager.

CMP   Comprehensive Metabolic Profile. A Medi-care-approved lab test for liver function and other testing. They specified the abbreviation as well. Similar to SMA-12.

CMS   Case Management Services. An organ-ization that provides case managers to SPMI patients.

CNS   Central Nervous System

c/o   Old medical abbreviation for "complains of." Also, in context, it means "care of" and "correctional officer."

Co.   County

CO   Correctional Officer

coc   Cocaine

COC   Contempt of Court. In context, it may be an abbreviation for 'cocaine.'

CON   Certificate of Need

condit   (or condits) Condition(s)

contrib (or contribs) Contribution(s)

CONUS Continental United States. A common acronym used in government service.

COPD   Chronic Obstructive Pulmonary Disease

CPAP   Continuous Positive Airway Pressure (a machine for obstructive sleep apnea)

CP&P   Child Protection and Permanency, (formerly the Division of Youth and Family Services: DYFS). An agency of state government. The name change followed a series of embarrassing lapses by the former DYFS.

CPS   Child Protective Services. An arm of a state government. In other states similar offices are CFS, CYS, DYFS etc.

CPR   Cardio-Pulmonary Resuscitation

CPTSD (or cPTSD) Complex PTSD. See DSO.

CPZ   chlorpromazine. Originally marketed as Thorazine (US) or Largactil (other places).

CR   Controlled Release. A form of medication where the release is spread out over time. In the cases of bupropion CR and lithium CR, the medications are designed to be released over 12 hours.

CRAF   Central Reception-Assignment Facility. A facility in a state prison system.

CSSD   Complex Somatic Symptom Disorder. A DSM-5 diagnosis.

CST   Child Study Team. Found in many schools. Always an indicator that the student had troubles.

CTE   Chronic Traumatic Encephalopathy, a degenerative brain disease caused by repeated undiagnosed head injuries, or concussions, often from playing football.

CYS   Children and Youth Services. An arm of a state government. In other states, similar offices are CPS, CFS, DYFS etc.

DA   Dopamine. A neurotransmitter involved with Parkinson's disease and psychosis. In non-medical contexts, district attorney.

DBD   Disruptive Behavior Disorder. DMDD is one kind of DBD.

DBT   Dialectical Behavior Therapy, a psychotherapy devised especially to meet the needs of people with Borderline Personality Disorder.

d/c   Depending on context, Discontinue (stop), or Discharge (as in to leave a unit or a facility).

Dec   Decanoate. An esterified form of decanoic acid. Seen with haloperidol decanoate and fluphenazine decanoate.

def   Defendant

decr   Decrease, decreased

del   Delusions

dep   Dependence. In other contexts dependent.

Dep   Deprecated. An abbreviation for Depakote, the original brand name of divalproex. Can be confused with 'dependence' and 'depression.' Use 'DVX' instead when you mean divalproex.

depr   Depressed, depression. Don't use 'dep.'

The reader may confuse that with 'Depakote,' 'dependence' or 'dependent.'

detox   Detoxification. The middle phase of the three-phase process that describes a person's disentanglement from dependence on a substance. These phases are **withdrawal**, **detox** and **rehabilitation**, or Rehab. They are nominally a week, a month and a year in duration.

devt   (or dev't) Development

DID   Dissociative Identity Disorder. The DSM-IV and DSM-5 term for multiple personality disorder.

diff   Different, to differ

difft   Different

dis   Disease, disorder. Deprecated. Use 'ds.'

disab   Disability, Disabled

disch   Discharge (as in to leave a facility), or a fluid that comes from the body

Disp: Disposition:

dissoc   Dissociate, dissociated, dissociative

dist   Disturbance. Outside medicine, it is short for 'distance' or 'distribution.'

distrib   Distributed, distribution.

disturb   Disturb, Disturbance, Disturbed

DJD   Degenerative Joint Disease

DMDD   Disruptive Mood Dysregulation Disorder. A diagnosis new for DSM-5 so that children do not get diagnosed "bipolar."

DMRD   Disruptive Mood Regulation Disorder. A diagnosis that includes DMDD.

D/O   disorder. Deprecated. See 'ds.'

DOA   Date of Arrest (in other contexts, Date of Admission or Dead on Arrival)

doc   Document

DOC   Date Of Commitment. The date an inmate was formally inducted into a correctional facility. In context, this may also mean Drug Of Choice or Department of Correction

doc'n   Documentation

DRG   Diagnostic Related Group. A Medicare payment system, where payment is based on the diagnosis and the length of stay associated with that diagnosis. Most psychiatry units are so-called "DRG-Exempt" where they are paid separately from the rest of the hospital. This means that any transfer from a DRG-exempt psychiatry unit to a medical unit requires a formal discharge and readmission. Likewise, a transfer from a medical unit to a DRG-exempt psychiatry unit requires a formal discharge and psychiatric admission. These formalities are dispensed with in the few DRG-Non-Exempt psychiatry units, so that transfers back and forth between hospital units are all part of the same admission.

ds   Disease, disorder. Preferred.

DSM   Diagnostic and Statistical Manual. Published by the APA, the American Psychiatric Association. We are now supposed to be using DSM-5.

DSO   Disturbances in Self-Organization—a seminal concept in the diagnosis of Complex PTSD (cPTSD): PTSD symptoms + DSO—affective dysregulation, negative self-concept and disturbances in relation-ships—that underlie a cPTSD diagnosis.

D/T   Due to

DUB   Dysfunctional Uterine Bleeding

DV   Domestic Violence

DVT   Deep Vein (or Venous) Thrombosis

DVX   Divalproex

dx   Diagnosis

DXM   Dextromethorphan

DYFS   Division of Youth and Family Services. A former arm of a state government. They changed the name to CP&P after DYFS was involved in some embarrassing lapses of supervision. In other states, similar offices are CFS, CYS etc.

E-x   Enlisted rank, all services. Actually the ranks go from E-1 to E-10 but you will almost never see anyone who had a rank higher than E-5.

EAP   Employee Assistance Program

ECT   Electroconvulsive Therapy. Shock treat-ment. A treatment for major depression and other serious psychiatric conditions.

ed   Education. Seen as the second part of "special ed."

ED   Emergency Dept. Depending on context, it can also mean Erectile Dysfunction or Emotionally Disturbed (a category in Special Ed).

EDP   Police acronym for Emotionally Disturbed Person

educ   Education, educational

EF   Executive function(s)

EHR   Electronic Healthcare Record. Also known as EMR.

emot   Emotion, emotional

EMDR   Eye Movement Desensitization and Reprocessing. EMDR is a successful treatment for PTSD and other problems in emotional development.

EMR   Electronic Medical Record. Another term for EHR.

EPS   Extrapyramidal system. Often used as a shortcut for EPS SE's (EPS side effects)

ER   Emergency Room. When appended to a medication name, Extended Release: a form of medication where the release is spread out over time. In the case of divalproex, the ER form is designed to release medication over 24 hours.

esp   Especially

Etoh   The ethylene molecule with a hydroxyl group (-OH). In chemistry, EtOH is the universal symbol for ethanol.

exec   Executive

F, (F)   Father. In typing, an uppercase F; in handwriting, an F with a circle around it.

FACT   Forensic Assertive Community Treatment program. A PACT team for felons.

FAS   Fetal Alcohol Syndrome (ICD-10 Q86)

FASD   Fetal Alcohol Spectrum Disorder (ICD-10 Q86). Person has a few physical features but not enough for a full diagnosis of FAS. See also ND-PAE (ICD-10 F88).

FB   Flashback. A reenactment of a trauma where the person experiences again the time, place and events of a trauma. Usually when people say "flashback" they mean "intrusive thought," where they re-experience a sight, sound or smell of a past trauma without actually feeling they are back there or reenacting it. In context, this may mean "Facebook."

FBS   Fasting Blood Sugar

FC   Foster Care

FNSD   Functional Neurological Symptom Disorder—a DSM-5 diagnosis that replaces conversion disorder.

FOI   Flight Of Ideas. A disorder in the FOT.

FOT   Flow Of Thought. A description of a subject's thinking as it transits from idea to idea.

FP   Family Practitioner

FPZ   Fluphenazine

FTA   Failure To Appear. In a jail chart this does not normally refer to the Fluorescent Treponemal Antibody component of the FTA-Abs test for syphilis.

FTD   Formal Thought Disorder—a disorder in the form of a patient's thinking. Outside jail, this may refer to a florist.

FTI   Free Thyroxine Index

FU   (also F/U) Follow-up

fx   Function. In a medical history, it might

mean 'fracture.'

GAD   Generalized Anxiety Disorder

GAF   Global Adaptive Functioning. The old Axis V in DSM-III and DSM-IV. An experiment that did not pan out, this was hard for clinicians to use, but gave the insurance companies a number they could latch onto. Thankfully, this "feature" was discarded in DSM-5.

GAS   Global Adaptation Scale. Same as GAF.

GERD   Gastroesophageal Reflux Disorder

GGP   Great Grandparents

GI   Gastro-Intestinal

gm   Gram

GM   In context, this may mean 'grandmother' or 'grand mal.' In non-medical circumstances, it can refer to General Motors, genetically modified, etc.

GP   Depending on context, General Practitioner, General Population, or Grandparents.

GSW   Gun Shot Wound

GTS   Gilles de la Tourette Syndrome. Same as TS

gtt   From Latin guttae, Drops

GU   Genitourinary

GWAS   Genome-Wide Association Study

h   hour

HA   Headache

HA1c   hemoglobin A1c, a marker for diabetes

HARP   Health And Recovery peer Program. A program for inmates to fight drug addiction, like SMART. In a medical chart, HARP does not refer to the Home Affordable

Refinance Program.

HAV   Hepatitis A Virus

hbA1c   hemoglobin A1c, a marker for diabetes

HBP   high blood pressure

HBV   Hepatitis B Virus

HCV   Hepatitis C Virus

HDL   High Density Lipoprotein

hgb   hemoglobin

hgbA1c   hemoglobin A1c, a marker for diabetes

Hg   Symbol for the element mercury

HI   Homicidal Ideation, head injury. In non-medical contexts, it is the address code for the state of Hawaii. See SI.

HIV   Human Immunodeficiency Virus

H&P   History and Physical

h/o   history of

hosp   hospital, hospitalization

HPI   History of the Present Illness (Only in NJ psychiatric hospitals does it mean Housing Preferences Index. This latter use should be avoided.)

HPV   Human Papilloma Virus

hr   hour

HR   Heart Rate

HS   An international medical abbreviation. From Latin for 'Hora Somnorum' or Hour of Sleep. In a social history, this means High School.

htn   hypertension

hx   history

IA   Internal Affairs. The office in a jail which investigates wrongdoing by CO's as well as arranging for the transfer of inmates with gang affiliations or other reasons to avoid general population.

IAD — Illness Anxiety Disorder—The DSM-5 term for hypochondriasis

ICD — International Classification of Diseases. Published by WHO the World Health Organization. The transition from ICD-9 to ICD-10 is now complete. Soon: ICD-11.

ICM — Intensive Case Manager. An intensive case manager may help a patient get to appointments, show up at court, fill out applications for Disability status, get medications etc. See CM and PACT.

ICMS — Intensive Case Management Services. An organization that provides ICM's to SPMI patients.

ID — Intellectual Disability. By Federal statue, this term replaces Mental Retardation (under "Rosa's Law"). In other contexts, ID stands for 'Identity' or 'Infectious Disease.'

IDD — Intellectual & Developmental Disability

IDR — Inmate Dining Room

IED — In context, it usually means Intermittent Explosive Disorder. Occasionally, it may mean 'Improvised Explosive Device' especially in the history of a veteran who is suffering from PTSD.

IEP — Individual Educational Plan

I&J — Insight and Judgment

IM — In context, this may mean 'inmate' or 'intramuscular.'

Imp: Impression:

inad   (or inadeq) Inadequate

incr   Increase(d)

indiv   Individual, individually

init   Initial, initially

inj   injured, injury

IPT   Interpersonal Therapy. A manualized form of structured psychotherapy.

IR   Immediate Release. A form of medication where the release of the chemical is not controlled or slowed. In other contexts it may mean Infra-Red.

IUP   Intrauterine Pregnancy

IV   intravenous

KOP   Keep On Person—a status where the patient or inmate keeps his or her medication on his or her person, or with his or her belongings.

LBP   Lower Back Pain

LDL   Low Density Lipoprotein

L   Liter

LD   Learning Disabled or Learning Disability

LDL   Low-Density Lipoprotein. A harmful lipoprotein.

LDX   lisdexamfetamine. A pro-drug that becomes amphetamine when metabolized.

LFT   Liver Function Tests or Testing

LMP   Last Menstrual Period

loc   Local, Localize(d), Located, Location

LOC   Loss Of Consciousness, as in a TBI or concussion

LSTL   Laparoscopic Tubal ligation

LWO   Living With Other. An older acronym, from the time when living unmarried with a domestic partner or "fiancée" was new.

m   minute (a measure of time). In a nonmedical context, meter.

M, (M) Mother. In typing, an uppercase M; in handwriting, an M with a circle around it.

MAOI   Monoamine Oxidase Inhibitor. The first group of antidepressants to be widely used. Because of the dietary restrictions needed to avoid hypertensive crises, these medications have mostly faded from use. They are still occasionally prescribed however, especially in cases of treatment-resistant depression (TRD), especially with true anxiety.

MAR   Medication Administration Record. This is a paper or electronic form that nurses use to record that a person received a medication that was ordered. In non-medical contexts, an abbreviation for the month of March.

MBD   Minimal Brain Dysfunction. An older term used to indicate ADHD. Not a current acronym.

mcg   Microgram; also written μg.

MDD   Major Depressive Disorder. This term has replaced 'melancholic depression.'

MDI   Manic-Depressive Illness or Manic-Depressive Insanity. The concept included melancholic depression (major depression) and what is now called bipolar disorder. Because it includes more than one illness, the term is no longer used. There are some who consider that all cases of major depression are cases of manic-depressive illness, though.

MDMA 3,4-methylenedioxy-methamphet–amine; Ecstasy, E-pill, Molly (though that last may refer to "bath salts").

med medical, medication, medicine

mg milligram

MH Mental Health

MI Myocardial Infarct. In some contexts, it may mean Mentally Ill.

MICA Mentally Ill Chemical Abuser. Used in Dual Diagnosis programs.

min Depending on context, minimum or minute.

MJ marijuana

mL milliliter

mmol millimole

MOS Military Occupational Specialty. Used in the Army. An example is 92B or Medic.

MPD Multiple Personality Disorder. A DSM-III term for what is now referred to as DID.

MR Mental Retardation. A now-obsolete term for intellectual disability, changed by Federal statute ("Rosa's Law") to ID.

MRE Most Recent Episode—as in DSM-IV/ICD-9 296.46 Bipolar Disorder, in Remission, MRE Manic. In the military, of course, MRE means 'Meal, Ready to Eat.'

MRI Magnetic Resonance Imaging or Image

MRSA Methicillin-Resistant Staphylococcus

Aureus

MSE   Mental Status Examination

MVA   Motor Vehicle Accident

MVP   Mitral Valve Prolapse

NA   Narcotics Anonymous

NAC   N-acetylcysteine

NB   Nota Bene

NCCHC National Commission on Correctional Healthcare. A review organization that is a lot more concerned about basic healthcare than the much-despised JCAHO.

ND-PAE Neurobehavioral Disorder-Prenatal Alcohol Exposure (ICD-10 F88). A DSM-5 term used when the prenatally alcohol-exposed subject does not have the physical stigmata needed to qualify for FASD or FAS (ICD-10 Q86). The diagnosis requires a history of more-than-minimal exposure to alcohol prenatally, deficits in neurocognitive functioning, self-regulation, and adaptive functioning.

NEC   Not Elsewhere Classified. The term that has replaced Not Otherwise Specified (NOS) in DSM-5.

neurol Neurological, neurology

NF   Non-Formulary

NIAAA   National Institute on Alcohol Abuse and Alcoholism. An agency of the Federal government.

NKDA   No Known Drug Allergy

NKMA   No Known Medication Allergy

nm   Nightmare. In context, it may refer to neuromuscular or nanometer.

NM   Neuromuscular. In context, New Mexico.

NMDA N-methyl-D-aspartate

NNH   Number Needed to Harm

NNT   Number Needed to Treat

nonform Non-formulary

NOS   Not Otherwise Specified. The classifier used in DSM-IV and ICD-10 to indicate a problem falling outside specific diagnoses. For example: F32.9 (311) Depression NOS. This diagnosis is used, because— due to the stress of a jail environment, and the unreliability of a history obtained from an inmate, who is often exaggerating to get drugs—we normally cannot differentiate between a major depression F32, F33 (296.2 or 296.3), a dysthymia F34.1 (300.4), an adjustment reaction with depressed mood F43.21 (309.0), or incarceration Z65.1 (a normal response to adverse circumstances, V62.5). The NOS classifier has been superseded in DSM-5 by NEC, but remains in ICD-10.

NP   Nurse Practitioner

NSAID Non-Steroidal Anti-Inflammatory Drug

NSSI   Non-Suicidal Self-Injury, a DSM-5 diagnosis. See also SIB.

ō   international medical abbreviation for 'nothing,' 'no,' 'not' or 'none'

O   When used as part of a SOAP note, Objective

OBS   Organic Brain Syndrome, used to describe episodes of dementia, delirium, intoxication, postictal confusion etc. Its main utility is to distinguish psychiatric from non-psychiatric physical psychosis. Embedded within the name is an uncertainty as to specific causation.

OCD   Obsessive-Compulsive Disorder

OCP   Obsessive-Compulsive Personality, which is *not* necessarily a disorder. After all, you would want your doctor or your accountant to pay obsessive attention to detail.

OD   From Latin, Oculus Dexter, right eye. In context, this may mean 'overdose.'

ODA   Orphan Drug Act

ODD   Oppositional Defiant Disorder. Beware using this. If you see a case of ODD, unpack it. Many cases of ODD are actually children who are reacting to an event like losing a parent, or getting sexually abused—in older terms, a reaction formation. Sometimes the children are labeled "bipolar" and receive medical attention, rather than counseling. A more neutral diagnosis would be DMDD, which was explicitly formulated to replace the widespread misdiagnosis of "bipolar" in children. Hopefully, in cases of disruptive children, you will look for signs of abuse or other causes of distress.

ODR   Officer Dining Room

OR   In context, Operating Room, Odds Ratio or the word 'OR' in uppercase.

OS   From Latin, Oculus Sinister, Left Eye

OSAS   Obstructive Sleep Apnea Syndrome

OTC   Over The Counter

OTH   Other Than Honorable. A type of discharge from one of the armed services. OTH discharged persons may still be eligible for VA care.

OTOH From online use: On The Other Hand.

OU   From Latin, Oculus Uterque, 'both eyes.'

ox   As in "pulse ox," a pulse oximeter, which is a clip-on device that noninvasively measures one's oxygen saturation.

Ox3   Oriented times three: oriented to person, place and time. Since many inmates intentionally ignore the calendar, thinking their time will pass more quickly, it often makes sense to ask an inmate to guess the date; or start with the year, then ask the month, then when during the month— early, middle or late.

Ψ   Psychiatric or Psychiatry, from the Greek letter psi.

p   [handwritten abbrev: small p with a line over it] international medical abbreviation for after, from Latin for 'post'

P   When used as part of a SOAP note, Plan.

PA   Physicians' Assistant. According to medical folklore this occupation came into being after the Vietnamese War to capture the experience of people who were combat medics there. Actually, the profession was proposed in 1961, based on how medics and corpsmen were trained for World War II. The first class started in 1965 with a bunch of former Navy corpsmen. In other contexts, it is short for Public Address or Pennsylvania.

PACT Psychiatric Assertive Community Treatment program or team. For the Severely and Persistently Mentally Ill (SPMI) population, a PACT team may bring medicines to the patient, assist the patient in taking the meds and take the patient for medical and other appointments. A PACT team is seen as a more intensive service than an ICM or a CM.

PAWS Post-Acute Withdrawal Syndrome A syndrome that often occurs during the rehabilitation phase of an addict's disentanglement from drugs.

PCP Phencyclidine ("angel dust"). In a jail context, it almost never refers to a Primary Care Provider or Pneumocystis Pneumonia.

PCO Polycystic Ovary disease. This can be a side effect of divalproex.

PCOS Polycystic Ovary Syndrome

PD (In context) Public Defender, Personality Disorder, Parkinson's Disease

PDNEC Personality Disorder NEC

PDNOS Personality Disorder NOS

PDR Physicians Desk Reference. A pre-Internet book that had all of the FDA warnings, the pill sizes and pictures of brand name medicines. There is still a website with those initials.

PE depending on context, Physical Examination or Pulmonary Embolism. In medical charts it does not refer to Physical Education.

PED   Prenatal Exposure to Drugs

PFC   Private First Class. E-3.

pgm   Program

PM   Afternoon

PMD   Premenstrual Dysphoria. See below.

PMDD   Premenstrual Dysphoric Disorder. This is a somewhat worse disorder than PMS, and is usually treated with SSRI's.

PMH   Past Medical History

PMS   Pre-Menstrual Syndrome

pna   Pneumonia

PO   Probation Officer or Parole Officer, depending on whether the inmate was on probation or parole. In other contexts, it may mean Police Officer or Per Oris – 'by mouth' in Latin.

POMR   Problem-Oriented Medical Record. An old movement. A reason to remember it is that it gave us the SOAP note.

PRN   International medical abbreviation, from Pro Re Nata, Latin for 'as the thing requires.'

p schiz   Paranoid schizophrenia

psychol   psychology, psychological, psychologist

PSD   Polysubstance Dependence

PTA   Prior To Admission. Used for hospitals. For jails use DOC, Date of Commitment. In a medical chart it does not refer to the Parent Teacher Association.

PTSD Post-Traumatic Stress Disorder

PUD Peptic Ulcer Disease. Peptic ulcers are now known to be caused by the bacterium *helicobacter pylori*, a spirochete. Although this condition can be exacerbated by stress, it is caused by *h pylori*, and can be cured with a two-week course of a four-medicine combination of a bismuth antacid, a proton pump inhibitor, metronidazole and an antibiotic. The restorative stage requires months of healing.

pvt Private soldier. E-2.

Q, Q's Question, Questions

QA Quality Assurance

QAM International medical abbreviation for 'each morning' or 'in the morning.'

QD International medical abbreviation for 'each day' or 'daily.' Contrary to some automated systems or facility policies, the original abbreviation does not mean 'each morning.'

QI Quality Improvement

QID international medical abbreviation for 'four times a day.'

QOD (do not use this) An informal alteration of QD—every day—that means 'every other day.' Easily confused with QD and QID. Deprecated.

QHS Deprecated. Use HS instead.

QPM (informal) Every afternoon.

RCT Randomized Controlled Trial

rec In context: Recommendation, Receive(d), Record(ed), Recreation rehab A rehabilitation facility. Although in a medical setting it often means a place to rebuild physical capacities, in a jail it usually means a place to recover from addiction. A drug rehab lasts 30 days or longer.

rel   Release. In context, Relative or Related.

relat   Relate(d), Relative, Relation, Relationship

RFA   Reason For Admission

RFR   Reason For Referral

rh   Rheumatoid, as in Rheumatoid Arthritis. In context, it may designate the Rh factor seen in blood types.

RIS   Responding to Internal Stimuli—visibly responding to hallucinations.

ROR   Released on Own Recognizance: released without bail.

ROS   Review of Systems

RSD   Reflex Sympathetic Dystrophy. You can use RSI for repetitive stress injury.

RSI   Repetitive Stress Injury

RTW Return to Work

Rx   Prescription, order (actually, it is an R with a crossed tail: ℞). In context, it can also stand for 'therapy' or 'therapeutic.'

rxn   reaction

s   [handwritten abbrev: small s with a line over it] International medical abbreviation for 'without,' from Latin 'sine.'

S   When used as part of a SOAP note, Subjective

S, (S) Sister. In typing, an uppercase S. In handwriting, an S with a circle around it.

sch School

schiz Schizophrenia or Schizophrenic

SCUT Schizophrenia, Chronic Undifferentiated Type. An old acronym, no longer used.

scz Schizophrenia or Schizophrenic

SE's Side effects

SES Socioeconomic Status

SI Suicidal Ideation. See HI.

SIB Self-Injurious Behavior. See NSSI.

SJS Stevens-Johnson Syndrome, a potentially fatal illness. When an inmate comes in taking lamotrigine you or the nurse must ask her when she last took the med. If more than four days have passed the nurse must NOT give it. Even if it was ordered within the 4-day time frame if she does not get the med within 4 days she MUST NOT RECEIVE IT. DISCON-TINUE IT. TEN is even more severe.

SJW St John's Wort. An herbal preparation used to treat depression. May conflict with SSRI antidepressants.

SMART Self-Management And Recovery Training. A program to combat addiction. Also called HARP.

SNRI Selective Norepinephrine-Serotonin Reuptake Inhibitors. A type of antidepressant. Analogous to SSRI.

SOAP Subjective Objective Assessment Plan—a structure for medical and surgical progress notes. See POMR.

soc social, socialize(d), society

S/P Status Post

Spec-4 Specialist-4. Equivalent to Corporal in combat arms. E-4.

Spec-5 Specialist-5. Equivalent to Sergeant in combat arms. E-5.

Spec ed (or Sp ed) Special Education. In days past, this referred to the special training given to the intellectually disabled. In more recent times, students with specific learning disabilities or behavior problems like ADHD receive special education. One question that comes up has been that boys outnumber girls by four- or five-to-one in special education programs.

SPMI Severely and Persistently Mentally Ill, usually referring to people highly disabled from schizophrenia.

SR Sustained release. The SR form of bupropion is designed to be released over twelve hours.

SSD Depending on context, either Somatic Symptom Disorder (a new DSM-5 diagnosis) or Social Security Disability, short for Social Security Disability Insurance. Outside of medicine, this means Solid State Drive, which is something that goes in your computer.

SSDI Social Security Disability Insurance. It will not be stopped on entry to jail.

SSI Supplemental Security Income—usually comes with attached Medicaid, but it *will* be stopped when the recipient is incarcerated, or hospitalized for a month or longer.

SSRI   Selective Serotonin Reuptake Inhibitor. A class of antidepressant medication.

SUD   Substance Use Disorder

SW   Suicide Watch. In context, Social Worker.

sx   Sign or Symptom, depending on context

sz   Seizure

T3   Tri-iodothyronine (liothyronine)

T4   Levothyroxine

TAH   Total Abdominal Hysterectomy

TB   Tuberculosis

TBI   Traumatic Brain Injury. In non-MH contexts, Tick Borne illness.

TCA   Tricyclic Antidepressant

TEN   Toxic Epidermal Necrolysis. Similar to but more severe than SJS.

TD   Tardive Dyskinesia

TG   Triglyceride

THC   Tetrahydrocannabinol, the active component of MJ.

TID   International medical abbreviation, from the Latin 'ter in die,' for 'three times a day.'

TLD   Temporolimbic Dysfunction or Temporal Limbic Dysfunction. Similar to TLE, but for the most part, without full-blown seizures. Dominated by impulsivity. Similar: Interictal Personality Disorder, Geschwind Syndrome.

TLE   Temporal Lobe Epilepsy

TR   Therapeutic Range

TRD   Treatment-Resistant Depression.

TS   Tourette Syndrome

TSH   Thyroid-Stimulating Hormone

tx   Treatment, Treating etc.

UC   Ulcerative Colitis. In context, University of California,

unspec Unspecified

URI   Upper Respiratory Infection

VA   Veterans Administration

VAH   Veterans Administration Hospital

VDL   Very low Density Lipoproteins

VH   Visual Hallucinations

vis   Visual. In context, Visible

VLDL   Very Low Density Lipoproteins

VNS   Vagus Nerve Stimulator

voc   Vocation, vocational. In context, may mean vocal, vocalize(d), vocalizing.

vocat   Vocation, vocational

VOP   Violation of Probation

VP   Violation of Parole

VS   Vital Signs

w/   With

WBC   White Blood Count

WL   Wait(ing) List

WNL   Within Normal Limits

w/o   Without

w/u   (or wu) Workup

XL   eXtra Long release. A form of medication where the release is spread out over time. The XL form of bupropion is designed to release the medication over 24 hours.

XR   eXtended Release. A form of medication where the release is spread out over time, usually 24 hours. For example, venlafaxine XR.

Y, yo   Years, Years Old

Appendix AL
Psychiatric Med Alerts

At your facility you may be required to continue psychiatric medications that have been verified by an outside pharmacy even before the inmate sees the inside shrink. Meds prescribed by psychiatrists in the community that are *not* prescribed in jail:

Benzodiazepines (Xanax, Klonopin etc.) - not used in jail.

Diphenhydramine (Benadryl) an anti–histamine which does not treat any psychiatric disorder. Diphenhydramine can be used as a substitute for benztropine. But when it is used by psychiatrists without an antipsychotic present, it is a drug. **Do not continue diphenhydramine unless it is accompanying an antipsychotic.**

Gabapentin (Neurontin) has no psychiatric indication. Physically it is used for seizures and pain, which are not psychiatric uses. **Do not continue a psychiatric prescription for this.**

Hydroxyzine (Atarax, Vistaril) is an antihistamine, which does not treat any psychiatric disorder. When used by psychiatrists, it is a drug. **Do not continue hydroxyzine unless it was prescribed by a medical specialist.**

Mirtazapine (Remeron) a sedating antidepressant. We use other antidepressants that are not sleep aids. **Do not continue it.**

Quetiapine (Seroquel) this has great abuse potential and many bad side effects. We use other antipsychotics. **Do not continue it.**

Topiramate (Topamax) has no psychiatric indication. It is used for seizures and migraines, which are not psychiatric uses. **Continue topiramate only if it was prescribed by a medical specialist, not a psychiatrist.**

Trazodone is most often used as a sleeping pill. **Do not continue it.**

Tricyclic Antidepressants (TCA's) are no longer used in jails by psych. **Do not reorder or continue them, even if verified.**

Take great care with these:

Lamotrigine (Lamictal) can cause Stevens-Johnson syndrome (SJS), a potentially fatal illness if lamotrigine is started abruptly or increased rapidly. When an inmate comes in taking Lamictal or lamotrigine, ask him or her when he or she last took it. Even if it was ordered within the 4-day time frame, if they don't get the med within 4 days DON'T GIVE IT. Discontinue it.

Bupropion (Wellbutrin)—the maximum amount of an immediate release or a crushed tab is 150mg per dose because of the risk of **seizures**. Do not give more than 150mg in a single dose unless it is bupropion SR or XL.

Bupropion is a much-abused substance. Consult with your protocols on whether it is banned at your jail or crushed when given.

Appendix CL
Psychiatric Med
Classification

When a medication is not used in jails do not continue it. Call the psychiatrist for an alternative medication.

Antipsychotic Meds (refer IM to psychiatrist)
    (Names in parentheses are trademarks)
    aripiprazole (Abilify)
    asenapine (Saphris)
    chlorpromazine (Thorazine)
    clozapine (Clozaril)
    fluphenazine (Prolixin)
    haloperidol (Haldol)
    iloperidone (Fanapt)
    olanzapine (Zyprexa)
    paliperidone (Invega)
    perphenazine (Trilafon)
    risperidone (Risperdal)
    ziprasidone (Geodon)

Antidepressant meds (refer IM to psychiatrist)

amitriptyline (Elavil) TCA. **Not used in jails.** May have been Rx'd for pain. Ask IM whether it is for pain, depression or sleep.
bupropion (Wellbutrin) Pay attention to plain (IR) vs CR vs XL forms. May be banned.

citalopram (Celexa) OK

desvenlafaxine (Pristiq) Not on formulary.

Desipramine (Norpramin) TCA. **Not used in jails.**

doxepin (Sinequan) TCA. **Not used in jails.**

duloxetine (Cymbalta) OK.

escitalopram (Lexapro) OK, if it is on the formulary. Otherwise, call the psychiatrist. Normally, the substitute is citalopram at twice the dose of escitalopram. Max escitalopram is 20mg.

fluoxetine (Prozac) OK.

imipramine (Tofranil) TCA. **Not used in jails.**

mirtazapine (Remeron) sleeping pill; not used in jails. **Do not continue it.**

nortriptyline (Aventyl, Pamelor) TCA, **not used in jails.**

paroxetine (Paxil) OK

sertraline (Zoloft) OK

trazodone (Desyrel) sleeping pill; not used in jails. **Do not continue it.**

venlafaxine (Effexor) OK

vilazodone (Viibryd) (not on formulary)

*Sleeping Pills (**not prescribed here**)*

chlorpromazine (Thorazine) also an anti–psychotic. Refer to psychiatrist.

diphenhydramine (Benadryl) an antihistamine; legitimate use only as alternate to Cogentin for EPS. Continue only if used with an antipsychotic. Otherwise, stop it.

doxepin (Sinequan) TCA. **Not used in jails.**

hydroxyzine (Atarax, Vistaril) antihistamine; no psychiatric use. **Do not continue it** if prescribed by a psychiatrist.

Mirtazapine (Remeron) antidepressant; soporific; **not used in jails**.

temazepam (Restoril) **benzodiazepine**

trazodone (Desyrel) sleeping pill; not used in jails. **Do not continue it.**

triazolam (Halcion) **benzodiazepine**. Known for prominent amnesic effects.

TCA (tricyclic antidepressant) **Not used in jails.** Fatal in OD.

zolpidem (Ambien) **Not used in jails.**

Anti-anxiety med on formulary here:
buspirone (Buspar) OK

Anti-anxiety meds
(drugs; not prescribed here)

alprazolam (Xanax) benzodiazepine

clonazepam (Klonopin) benzodiazepine

diphenhydramine (Benadryl) antihistamine; legit use only as alternate to Cogentin for EPS. Continue only if used with an antipsychotic.

hydroxyzine (Atarax , Vistaril) antihistamine; not used here for anxiety.

lorazepam (Ativan) benzodiazepine

Anti-Convulsants (dual-use; may also be for seizures, pain, headaches)

carbamazepine (Tegretol) may be for medical or psych; **OK if for psych**

divalproex (Depakote) may be for medical or psych; **OK if for psych**

gabapentin (Neurontin) NO psychiatric use.

lamotrigine (Lamictal) may be for medical or psych; **OK if for psych, but unsafe if more than four days between doses.**

oxcarbazepine (Trileptal) may be for medical or psych; **OK if for psych**.

topiramate (Topamax) NO psychiatric use.

Anti-EPS and Restlessness-Reducing Meds

Benztropine (Cogentin) anti-parkinsonian anti-EPS. OK

clonidine (Catapress) antihypertensive + anti-ADHD; **not used by psychiatrists in jails**.

propranolol (Inderal) antihypertensive + anti-akathisia + anti-anxiety; **not used by psych-iatrists in jails**.

trihexyphenidyl (Artane) anti-parkinsonian + anti-EPS. OK

Anti-PTSD med:

prazosin (Minipress) antihypertensive + anti-PTSD; **not used by psychiatrists in jails**.

Not Used in Jails

amphetamine (Adderall) amphetamine salts
armodafinil (Nuvigil)
dextroamphetamine (Dexedrine)
dexmethylphenidate (Focalin)
methamphetamine (Desoxyn)
methylphenidate (Ritalin)
modafinil (Provigil)
Any opiate (no psychiatric indications)
Any benzodiazepine

Appendix D
Dissociative Identity Disorder

Dissociative Identity Disorder (DID) is a highly controversial topic. A number of our colleagues do not believe it exists. You might be one of these colleagues. If so, you can skip this appendix.

After 30 years dealing with known dissociative identity disorder, I have come to the conclusion that the most helpful metaphor for treatment is to liken DID to an addiction. DID appears to arise when a person—usually a very young person—is exposed to more trauma than she believes she can endure. So the victim hypnotizes herself into not being present. She dissociates. Psychologically, she has escaped. She is not there. See the end of the movie *Brazil* for an example.

What remains may become . . . something. Perhaps in some cases, the victim of the trauma personifies the dissociated state. The alternate personality can take over consciousness of the traumatized person. She can even take a name.

What reason would the traumatized victim have for keeping an alternate personality (called an alter) around? The alter would be useful when —and there is usually a when—the abuse is repeated. Eventually the victim creates more and more alters. Initially, the causes were traumas. After a time, the causes are more trivial. One patient of mine, for example, did not like to write checks. So she would dissociate, and leave the check writing to an alter, the responsible one.

Victims are like drug addicts, but younger. Just as adult drug addicts seem like adolescents, the primary personalities of DID people seem like children (the alters, OTOH, are usually mature-seeming). In both cases, the apparent age reflects the time when they quit growing up and started to depend on something or someone else to cope with their problems.

For the primary personalities of people with DID, the process of dissociation is their escape from reality. Rather than grapple with an issue and develop the requisite coping skills, people with DID dissociate and let their alters cope with the situation. Or they dissociate and create a new alter to cope with the situation. The primary personality never herself copes with trouble.

For this reason, the alters come to despise their primary personality. When they are not in control, the alters are experienced by the primary as derogatory voices. The primaries often know their alters as derogatory voices with names attached to the voices. Sometimes, they are not consciously aware of the dissociative process. In one case this was so extreme that a patient was convinced that space aliens were coming in and moving her things around while she slept.

Diagnosis of DID

Diagnosing DID requires that you have an index of suspicion. After all, you don't normally go through and ask a person if she ever finds herself wearing makeup she does not remember putting on, wearing clothes she does not remember putting on, having her hair in hairdos she does not recall. You don't normally ask someone if she has found herself in places she does not remember going to; whether strangers recognize her; whether strangers call her by strange names. Usually you will come to this suspicion by getting a history of extreme serial abuse. Or you will have a history that suddenly seems inexplicably bland.

Sometimes a person will switch from a distressed primary to a well composed alter. If you recognize the transition, you can then ask questions involving the dissociative process.

Know, however, that this is a relatively easy diagnosis to fake. Luckily, there is no chemical treatment for DID. As with PTSD, you can treat a concomitant depression. But other than that, there is no chemical for the condition.

Treatment of DID

Experts on DID have their own approaches to treating cases of DID. I have found these approaches are too time-consuming for busy professionals. Also, when I have observed others

trying to emulate them, I have observed unfortunate outcomes. I have fallen back on the "Coaching
Method" of DID treatment.

In essence, we coach the person with DID to
treat herself. The treatment itself is composed of
three phases: the victim will get back her Present,
get back her Past and get back her Pieces.

Sometimes, the easiest things to say are the
hardest things to do.

Present The function of DID in a patient's
ecosystem is to maintain homeostasis. Whenever
the primary confronts a situation she does not
know how to handle, she dissociates and an alter
takes over. You can imagine how the alters feel
about this behavior. Whenever the going gets
tough, the primary runs away, scurrying for
cover, leaving the alters to figure out how to deal
with the difficulty. Often the alter fights, since she
knows how to do that.

Each alter views the world in tunnel vision,
seeing the problem through her own narrow
point of view. Since she sees the problem narrowly, she sees the solution narrowly. After all, she
was probably created to deal with a specific
circumstance the primary personality found to be
difficult. Finding an alter who is tailored to fighting situations is common, for example. Fun-loving
and seductive alters are often present, as well.

One key is talking to the alters through the
primary personality. Although you invite the
alters to listen in, you explain what follows to the
primary personality. In essence, you ask the
alters to "Just Say No to dissociation" (the quote

will sound familiar to those who were present in the 1980's fight against drug use). Alters will refrain from taking over consciousness. While alters may assist the primary and while they may engage in "co-consciousness" to help the primary—figuratively whispering guidance in her ear—they may not take over.

From now on, the primary personality must be in charge of her own body 24/7 while she is awake. The alters may speak to her through intrapsychic voices, and tell her that they agree to this. She can then relay their assents to the therapist. However, none of them may be allowed to take over and speak directly to the therapist. The therapist must model keeping the primary personality in the here-and-now.

Sometimes you can tell when an alter has taken over. Often it is a change in demeanor. Feel free to ask who you are speaking to. If the person talking to you is an alter, ask her to step back and leave the primary in charge.

The goal is that the primary should gain strength by dealing with difficulties herself. In a way, this is fitting punishment: she must now do what she has always called upon alters to do. They must not let her dissociate. As the primary personality becomes stronger, the alters will have less reason to despise her. This will take time, but an inmate has nothing but time.

Past At times of their own choosing, alters can share with the primary pieces of what they are hiding from her. They should start with glimpses that are a few seconds in duration. They know how much their primary can tolerate. They can give her the past in bits and pieces, all in fragments their primary can handle.

As the primary personality becomes stronger through the actions of the alters in giving her back her Present, she will be able to handle larger and longer glimpses of her past traumas. Note that the alters decide when the primary can deal with what they have been hiding from her. The therapist never forces this. In fact, this process goes on without the intervention of the therapist. The therapist is a coach here, not directly involved in the process.

Pieces At some point various alters will work themselves out of a job. No longer will they be taking over from the primary: she will be strong enough to handle her troubles on her own. No longer will they be hiding past traumas from the primary: they will have unveiled them all. At this juncture, the alter may choose to join the primary so they are a joint personality.

Before fusing personalities, a person with DID looks at the world the way an insect does, with each alter and the primary seeing the world through her own little tunnel. But by fusing personalities, the primary and an alter enlarge their vision, seeing more like a mammal and less like an insect. But the important point here is that the alter chooses when to merge with the primary. No one is pushing her to merge. This is a key mistake that therapists make in treating cases of DID. Fusion is not only a voluntary process, it must occur at the time and place of the alter's choosing. Any other course would feel too much like abuse.

Gender and DID

After years of dealing with cases of DID I have observed that male patients seem to have fewer alters than female patients. Females seem to have many alters. They also seem to have fragments of alters. Sometime alters are no more than a face. This may reflect the greater victimization of females in all societies. This may reflect the greater rebelliousness found in many males.

Blame in DID

What one alter does, the whole body does. As a factual matter, the whole body gets the blame and the whole body goes to jail. So it **is** fair for the primary to get locked up in a jail for something her alter did—without the primary even 'knowing' what it was. This "you're all in it together" concept is what makes a patient see that her best interest lies in conquering dissociation to achieve fusion. The process is much like recovery from drug addiction.

Fake DID

Some inmates will try to fake DID. Perhaps the most common reason is to get you to prescribe drugs or antipsychotic meds as quasi-drugs. Luckily, we do not prescribe comfort pills.

Some inmates are faking a case of multiple personality because they think they can escape responsibility for their crimes. As long as you stay out of forensic psychiatry, you can leave that concern to the forensic consultant and the judge.

Personality and DID

When dealing with DID, remember "Hume's Rule" about this condition: "multiple personality disorder means multiple *borderline* personality disorder."

Appendix E
EHR (Electronic Health Record)

One thing has happened that has changed the face of medical practice: the electronic medical record. Now, management pays more than $100 an hour to a physician to type far more slowly than a $12/hour typist. Go figure.

But we are stuck with our systems, and they differ. For example, one of the EMR systems I have used allows a text replacement feature, which can expand certain letter combinations. That allows me to type in a few letters, and get expanded portions of history or MSE's; then complete the notes by adding details, or trim them by cutting words; sometimes details are added with more use of the text replacement feature. All this allows me to be far more productive.

Some EMR systems operate on your browser. This has the advantage of being accessible via the Internet. This makes telepsych possible. But there is no text replacement ready to make typing quicker, and you can lose your work with an errant keystroke. In such cases, you may want to have the whole history saved in a desktop document; it can be copied from there and pasted into the clinical record. But then it requires pruning some details and filling in others.

Examples for text replacement:

fu =   "IM seen for routine follow-up. Current
        medication order:"
br =   "Born and raised in"
pmh = "PMH:" or "Past Medical History:"
mse = "MSE: Alert, jiggling feet leg, fidgeting;
otherwise normoactive. Euthymic Anxious Angry
mood with broad normally responsive congruent
subdued blunted affect and normal irritable
expansive demeanor. Flow of thought normal:
non-pressured, goal-directed, relevant and
logical. No delusions elicited. Not responding to
internal stimuli. Wants to live. Denies homicidal
ideation. Denies current voices. Denies suicidal
ideation. Fully oriented. Memory grossly intact.
Intellectual functioning not grossly impaired.
Insight and judgment fair." [This would have
more text, but the text replacement field is
limited]
sm =   "Smiles and laughs spontaneously."
w/   "with"
etc.

In this interface, since automatic correction is
not available, you basically have to program in
any common mistypings: e.g.—currnet = current
etc.

These shortcuts really speed up typing.

The following may or may not speed up your typing. They are automatic text for diagnoses:

f88	=	"F88 ND-PAE"
f90	=	"F90 ADHD"
z65.1	=	"Z65.1 Incarceration"

There is another function in an EMR app where you can bring up and paste into the record a list of current meds prior to the inmate being seen, and again a list of meds after the inmate is seen. Having a list of meds in front of you allows you to know what your patient is getting. Having a list of meds after you have made changes allows you to review what the inmate will be getting. If you have made a mistake, you have a chance to correct it before you make the record final.

In the browser-based EHR, there may be a list of meds that is visible. You can copy it, and paste it into your record. I recommend you do so. It is a snapshot of the meds that were current when you were seeing the inmate. This can be invaluable in going back to see what an inmate was taking at a time when he was doing well or poorly.

It is also a good idea to make a formal diagnosis when you see a patient for the first time. It may help you to list the diagnoses in order of their appearance. For example:

"dx (3/4/16; updated 5/1/19):

F90	ADHD
F43.12	chronic PTSD (from childhood)
F60.3	Borderline Personality Disorder
F11.2	Opiate dependence
F13.2	Iatrogenic BZD dependence
-----	s/p TBI with seizures"

You can then take the whole block of text and paste it into each progress note. This will serve as a reminder of just what you are treating. It is dated, to show when the symptoms supporting the diagnosis were collected. Additional diagnoses should include a date in parentheses to show when that diagnosis was added; in other words, where to find the report of the supporting symptoms.

You can even have a skeleton workup saved as a block, so you can add details and prune as needed. It saves typing.

If your EHR has a price function built in, check to make sure its database is up to date. If it is, you will be able to learn the true cost of the medications you are prescribing. That is a very helpful function.

See also Chapter 9.

Appendix G
Glossary

(For 'Street Talk' see the next section of this Appendix.)

Akathisia Motor restlessness. Greek for 'no chair' or not sitting. It is a form of restlessness where the afflicted person only feels comfortable when he is pacing. It can accompany antipsychotics, especially first-generation antipsychotics but also second-generation antipsychotics. When combined with akinesia, it can be excruciating, causing the afflicted patient to want to get up and pace, yet be unable to do so.

Akinesia This is a form of psychic paralysis that can accompany antipsychotics, especially first-generation antipsychotics. When combined with akathisia, it can be excruciating, causing the afflicted patient to want to get up and pace, yet be unable to do so.

Alter Alternate Personality, as seen in Dissociative Identity Disorder (see Appendix D).

Audio-Video Electronic terms, not used (deprecated) in medicine.

Auditory and Visual Human sensory perceptions; terms used (preferred) in medicine.

Character Disorder is no longer used. The term once described people whose distress arose from personality disorders—from their characters; hence the term.

Comfort Pill A pill which can be used by anyone, not just people suffering from a mental illness. Usually these are soporific chemicals. See discussion under 'Drugs,' below.

Depression is an illness, not a mood state. A normal person will feel down, unhappy, sad, upset when things don't go his way. Maybe he has trouble sleeping. It may be from ADHD (see Appendix H), or he is merely worried. He may not have the mental illness diagnosed as 'depression.' See also 'Depression' in 'Street Talk' below.

Detox This stands for the detoxification phase of disentanglement from a substance. It follows withdrawal, precedes rehab, and is nominally a month in duration.

Discontinuation Syndrome This is distinct from a Withdrawal Syndrome, in that although you will feel like you want to die, it will not kill you. A withdrawal syndrome may kill you.

A discontinuation syndrome makes you feel like you have the flu, with malaise, sleeplessness, nausea, imbalance, hyperarousal, even electric shocks in the brain.

You see this most often when someone suddenly stops venlafaxine or paroxetine, but you can see it with citalopram and sertraline. Treat this by restarting the med. Prevent a recurrence by tapering the dose or starting another SSRI at full dose.

Drugs As used in this book, the term 'drug' is used to describe any chemical which has psycho-active properties in normal people. Its effects are not confined to people with mental illness, so it is not a medication. Sometimes a chemical can be both a drug and a medicine. Tricyclic antidepressants are the most prominent example. But TCA's should not be used in jails because they can be deadly in overdose and inmates will overdose themselves chasing the drug effects of these chemicals. The safest policy is No Drugs.

Still need convincing? In the 1970's we gave our post-op patients hydroxyzine to reduce their need for opiates. Those patients were not mentally ill. As a side note, I will observe that doctors were still minimizing the use of opiates in those days, trying to avoid producing iatrogenic opioid addicts. This was before the days of pain scales, etc. In fact, opiate withdrawal is often managed with hydroxyzine.

Dystonia is a cramping that can affect one muscle or the whole body. It can even cause a body to twist or a tongue to thrust out. Dystonias are very uncomfortable, even painful. Although there can be other causes, most often psychiatrists see this as an EPS side effect of antipsychotics. You treat this with benztropine or diphenhydramine.

Instrumental behavior—doing something to get something.

Long Term Rehab is the final phase someone's disentanglement from a substance. It may be lifelong, and it is all about learning to live without substances.

Medicines Also known as '**medications**.' These are chemicals used to treat medical and mental illnesses. Think SSRI.

Oculogyric Crisis is when the eyes roll up. It is a form of dystonia, a side effect of antipsychotic meds.

Reactive behavior—acting in response to a stressor, often without thinking first.

Rehab is short for rehabilitation and is the penultimate phase of someone's disentanglement from a substance. This phase nominally lasts a year.

Sign is something you see.

Symptom is something a person reports.

Video Electronics term. Do not use it.

Visual Use this instead.

Vorbeireden is a German word that means 'talking past the point.' A person knows the right answer but deliberately gives a wrong answer. When you ask someone the date and they give you a date that is 13 months from now, that is vorbeireden. This is also called 'the syndrome of approximate answers.' You will usually see it when an inmate is trying to appear crazy, but not *too* crazy. It is instrumental behavior.

Withdrawal is an episode of elevated vital signs (and sometimes seizures) that follows the stopping of various drugs. It precedes the detoxification phase. Often detox programs will not let an addict in until the withdrawal is done.

Withdrawal can lead to death, so withdrawal from alcohol and benzodiazepines is usually ameliorated with oral chlordiazepoxide. Often, opiate withdrawal is ameliorated with hydroxyzine. Clonidine is better for this purpose, but in a jail, the doctor is often not on site; so because of the possibility of serious hypotension, clonidine is not commonly used for opiate withdrawal in a jail.

Street Talk for Shrinks

(In previous editions, this section came at the end of Chapter 2.)

For you to get ready for the inmate population you need hear what they are saying to you. You have to learn to unpack words in common use. They are often words borrowed from psychiatric terms without a complete understanding of their true meaning. If you merely accept at face value the words inmates tell you, you may miss what they mean.

"Anti-Social" When our people use this term to describe their behavior, they usually mean social withdrawal—*asocial*, not anti–social behavior like robbery and such. They don't think of themselves as criminal, but a fair amount of them have social phobia and hence social withdrawal. Since the term 'antisocial' is often flung about in reference to them or people they know, they use "anti-social" to mean social withdrawal.

"Anxious" (See also Chapter 5.) The term *anxiety* is often used with *nervous*. Anxiety in psychiatry is a form of alarm. People with social phobia and panic disorder have anxiety, for example. But when used on the street, "anxiety" can be the motor restlessness of ADHD; a feeling of eager anticipation; irritability; or a physical tremor—the person infers inner fear, but the symptom may reflect that, or essential tremor, or the tremor of withdrawal, or a side effect of medication. In other words, the word "anxiety" could mean a number of things to a layperson (the list of potentials was not exhaustive) so what the inmate means when she says she is "anxious" must be determined each time, not assumed.

"Attorney" People in this stratum often do not recognize that public attorneys/defenders are attorneys. They don't even know the DA or prosecutor is an attorney. What they mean when they say "attorney" is 'private defense attorney.'

"Blackout" This term is used to add drama to the description of someone acting out his rage. Supposedly a person would be so angry that he recollected nothing of what had occurred—hence "blackout." Now, by extension, it has come to mean any angry acting out, whether the angry actor remembers it or not. It is possible that the person was so enraged that he dissociated, or had a partial complex seizure. But the only way to know is to inquire of the inmate and record the answers (otherwise known as unpacking the term).

The use of the 'blackout' to describe an episode of heavy drinking is an older concept, apparently unknown to inmates today.

"Bipolar" When someone has a labile mood or emotional dysregulation, she is said to have "mood swings," and thus is "bipolar." The incidence of true bipolar disorder in the community is about 2%, but the diagnosis is the norm for inmates. Why? If you have a depressed patient insured under managed care, you will have to justify keeping her in your treatment. The care manager wants to know why you haven't cured the patient and moved her on. On the other hand, nobody bothers you if your patient carries a diagnosis of 'bipolar disorder.' Hm. If you are a rehab facility, you can detox a person once or maybe twice under his insurance, but for further coverage, you will need a second diagnosis, a psychiatric one. Maybe your patient must have a "dual diagnosis" to qualify for care. If your patient has a labile mood from absence of substances she has an unstable mood. Unstable mood? Must be "mood swings," justifying a diagnosis of "bipolar disorder." And this justifies reimbursement by the insurance company. After all, bipolar disorder is a biological and hereditary psychiatric disorder.

Inmates have been told they are "bipolar" when they have an exaggerated response to normal events—in other words, emotional dysregulation. Their normal lifestyle is such that when they run into uncomfortable events like someone dying or something else bad happening, they take a pill, use a drug or drink alcohol. They don't expect to feel unhappy when events call for feeling unhappy. Actually, they can't cope with good news any better than bad. Good times or bad times, every event produces "mood swings" which must be dampened by drugs; if they cannot obtain prescribed drugs they will "self-medicate." Whatever, the fact that they have "mood swings" means they "have bipolar." Worse, their aunt or mother was diagnosed "bipolar," which solidifies it, since everybody knows it is hereditary. They may say their moods swing spontaneously, but they do not notice they are responding to something.

"**Depressed**" This usually means *unhappy* on the street. Any "stress" can make people un-happy, even a normal response to a stressor; so people become "depressed," which to them is a normal feeling, an emotional response. Do not believe that people automatically can distinguish between unhappiness and depression. Some can, but most jailbirds cannot—or will not—tell the difference. And even if they can, they will say they are "depressed," fishing for drugs.

"**Flashback**" This can refer to a symptom of PTSD. But another older use for the term is an LSD flashback. The term actually refers to the dramatic re-experiencing and reenactment of traumatic events by Vietnam War veterans—a sign identified with PTSD.

Usually, inmates mean they are experiencing intrusive thoughts when they use this word. But they occasionally use this term correctly, as a description of a literal re-experiencing of a traum-atic event. As usual, the term needs unpacking.

"**Manic**" If you have ever taken care of true bipolars, you may remember seeing real manic patients. But I have had inmates sitting quietly in front of me telling me they were in the midst of a manic episode. Often inmates will use the word to describe ADHD symptoms or the irritability that can accompany withdrawal. Obviously, they are not manic. Ask them to delineate their problems, but **do not poll them on symptoms**. Let them explain their symptoms in their own words. If you ask them about specific symptoms, you are educating them about the issues that interest psychiatrists. They treasure information like that.

"**Mood Swings**" This phrase is used to refer to a labile mood. The term 'mood swing' was coined to describe an often-dramatic change observed when a depressed person shifted to a full-blown manic episode, usually within hours. As used on the street, the term "mood swings" is used to describe labile moods, usually emotional dysregulation, with moods changing in seconds, and provides the excuse needed for a diagnosis of "bipolar disorder." Emotional dysregulation is an old observation in neurotic depression, border-line personality disorder and other "character disorders." In essence, you have an exaggerated response to a stressor, good or bad. The labile mood described in the colloquial term "mood swings" may also result from a depression, with its frequently intermittent symptoms. However you find it, the term must be unpacked to derive any useful data from it.

"Night Terrors" This is a straight misuse, where people on the street have hijacked a useful medical term to describe nightmares or vivid dreams. A night terror is actually a neurologic process that occurs during the non-REM sleep of young children. When an inmate uses the term, she means she is having nightmares, a part of REM sleep. She might not even be having a recurring dream. Vivid dreams have been described as a feature of TCA's, SSRI's and SNRI's. Vivid dreams are also a common feature of drug withdrawal. But the inmate complaining of "night terrors" may simply be under some stress. As usual, when an inmate uses a technical term, what she means by the term must be explored.

"Panic Attacks" A panic attack is dramatic and often involves a "Code Blue" or similar medical intervention. Or it could involve lesser drama. Leaving aside false "panic attacks" (I once had a patient sit next to my desk and calmly state that she was in the middle of a panic attack), what inmates usually mean is that they had a fearful response to adrenaline. Here I tell them to look at their hands—usually their palms are pink or the beds beneath their fingernails are pink. As long as that is true, they are getting plenty of air—no matter how short of breath they feel.

Although these naïve waifs are taught how to put a condom on a banana in health class, they learn nothing of human physiology. There are times I tell them that the body responds to danger. It must prepare you to fight or flee. How does it do that? It gets the muscles primed with oxygen. How does that happen? First you bring air into your lungs, where the oxygen gets into your blood. Then your heart pumps it out to the muscles. How does that feel? First, you feel air hunger—you feel short of breath—so you will pull in extra air to charge up the blood in your lungs. Then your heart pounds hard to move that blood. You can feel your heart doing that. Then you feel hot all over as the blood dumps oxygen off on your muscles. So when you feel short of breath and your heart is pounding, your body is behaving *normally* in a threatening situation. And jail is a threatening situation.

"**Paranoid**" Paranoia is a fear of people and forces you cannot see—forces and people that wish to do you harm. This is a psychotic process and is relatively unusual. Social phobia is much more common. Social phobia is so common that AA and NA unconsciously have designed their programs to combat it. Social phobia is the fear of the people you see before you. As one inmate said "I feel nervous, like all the attention's on me." A socially phobic person will get more nervous the closer he or she gets to a group of five to forty people, especially strangers. She feels they are judging her. He feels they are looking down on him, plotting against him or intending him harm. Inmates may say "paranoid" to mean true paranoia, but they usually mean to say that something makes them nervous. Usually, this something is groups of people, and they have social phobia, not psychosis. Sometimes they have social phobia as part of PTSD. As usual, you must unpack their use of the word to know if they are truly paranoid, or merely have social phobia, or some other form of anxiety.

BTW: AA and NA put their members in front of groups to talk of their experiences. They force their members to confront groups of people, often strangers. This is, of course, counterphobic conditioning. Psychologists will recognize the systemic exposure of extinction therapy.

"Prosecutor and Public Defender" Jail-going people often do not recognize that DA's and prosecutors are attorneys. They don't even know that public defenders are attorneys. What they mean when they say "attorney" is 'private attorney.'

"Psych pill" Often an inmate will take an antidepressant or an ADHD med and not believe that this was a "psych" med. "Psych meds" in this view are antipsychotic drugs. Be sure to unpack what the inmate means when she dumps this load in her history. In fact, if she is taking an antipsychotic for sleep or "anxiety" she might have a dystonic reaction and call it a "seizure" (see).

"Racing Thoughts" The term 'racing thoughts' was used to describe one of the signs—not a symptom—of the psychomotor acceleration most often seen in mania. From the manic patient's perspective we are slowed down; the patient believes he is functioning at a normal rate. What "racing thoughts" means on the street is one of crowded thinking; most often it is one of the symptoms of ADHD, but it could refer to the sense of things going out of control that anxious (fearful) people have, or even depressive ruminations. Again, you must unpack the term to find out what the inmate means when she uses it.

"Seizure" Often inmates will say they have a history of "seizures" when they have had nothing of the sort. When inmates have episodes of dystonia or oculogyric crises they will call them "seizures." You must inquire in some detail about these reported events, so you are sure they have seizures and not episodes of acute EPS side effects. Intellectually disabled people, for example, might not know that what they have been taking was a "psych pill."

"Self-medicating" Psychiatry is known in the substance abuse treatment community as being a profession of enablers. But our greatest act of enabling substance abusers is the idea that substance abusers are "self-medicating." The concept is permission-giving for addiction and such concepts as "addiction substitutes." Getting intoxicated by drinking alcohol and/or using drugs is all about getting high. It might also be a way to avoid bad feelings, of hiding from one's troubles. People may have painful feelings, and using substances covers those feelings up for a time. But using substances is a cover, not a cure.

Substances are not any kind of medication. In fact, even some medications are drugs, and some medicines used for side effects are drugs. It is no accident that drug addicts, alcoholics and people with ADHD and BPD ask for benzodiazepines, chlorpromazine, doxepin, gabapentin, hydroxyzine, quetiapine, diphenhydramine, mirtazapine, thioridazine and trazodone: they simply do not want to experience life raw, as it is. But it is most important that they do so.

Appendix H
ADHD

For fifteen years, I have been asking the same screening questions of all people I see: Did you have trouble sitting still or paying attention when you were young? If the person says yes, I ask two more questions: Did you have trouble getting to sleep at night, thinking about everything in the world, with racing thoughts? Were you impulsive, doing stuff suddenly, without thinking about it first? Among hospital consultations the rate for getting a Yes to three or four questions was around 5%. At a state hospital, the rate was between 5% and 10%. Among jail populations, the positivity for 3 or 4 questions ranges from 85% to 95%, at a stable rate for each jail, regardless of when the inmate was born. Studies of jail populations have shown a formal diagnostic rate of 60%. Whatever the number, more than half of your population will have ADHD, so ADHD complaints will be common.

ADHD has been misnamed. There is no deficit of attention in ADHD, for example. If you have seen someone with ADHD ensconced in a video game he likes, for example, just try getting his attention. Or see if you can get an ADD patient away from a book she really likes. These are difficult things to do. ADHD is the I'll-Pay-Attention-To-What-I-Want-To-Pay-Attention-To Disorder. Conversely, ADHD is the I-Won't-Pay-Attention-To-What-You-Want-Me-To-Pay-Attention-To disorder. Or you could call it the I-Can't-Sit-Still disorder. Depending on how you define it, the prevalence is somewhere between one in seven (loosely defined ADHD) and one in 25 (tightly defined ADHD) in the population at large. This phenomenon of lessened prevalence as one tightens the criteria suggests that ADHD is one end of a bell curve with normals in the middle at the high point.

If ADHD is simply a variant of normal, it would be like diagnosing "tallness disorder" in the population. Just as the person who is taller than a doorframe must duck his head to get through without bruising himself, someone with ADHD must make adaptations to civilized society to get through life. Remember the old saying that "Idle hands are the Devil's workshop?" ADHD people must keep busy doing constructive things, or they may find themselves doing destructive things.

Another thing: brain differences can be measured in individuals, but a person's height can also be measured. Physical signs, then, do not necessarily mean someone is ill.

First and foremost, ADHD people seem to have memory difficulties. There are many things they simply don't retain. Yet studies show that—suitably motivated—they have normal memories. It turns out that the attention and memory are issues of executive functioning. As we have already noted, ADHD people can pay attention to things they find intrinsically interesting. But even they can't make themselves pay attention to something they are not interested in, much less something *you* want them to learn.

ADHD people describe thinking of something else while you are talking to them. Their minds "wander all over the place." They are easily distracted. The phrase "Look! A squirrel!" comes to mind.

Sleep What bothers an ADHD person the most is "I can't turn my mind off" at night. They think about "everything" at night. They complain of "racing thoughts" that begin just as soon as they lie down. This is almost a universal complaint among ADHD people. At home, they chase sleep with drugs and alcohol or stay up late and get up late. In jail, they can prevail on psychiatrists to give them legal drugs—soporific substances that can be ordered. In the ADHD community, this phenomenon is often treated with clonidine or with a small amount of methylphenidate at night. The advantage of using these medications is the physician is treating the ADHD symptoms to achieve sleep.

Since the inmate is thinking about everything while he is awaiting sleep, you can tell him he is dreaming while he is awake, thinking things through and solving problems. Since the purpose of dreaming is to sort through issues, he is accomplishing those very goals by lying awake and thinking. If he gets up in the morning and stays awake all day (thus observing good sleep hygiene) then lies down and lets his body rest at night, his body will steal the sleep it needs. This notion of stealing fits into the criminal mindset.

Often an inmate will complain that he is finally feeling tired and ready for sleep when the morning comes; then he sleeps through the morning. He might benefit from sleep hygiene.

But he simply may not need much sleep. It is a common pattern that people with ADHD may short themselves on sleep for five or six days then use the weekend to catch up, occasionally sleeping 24 hours through. Or maybe he is like Babe Ruth. In a recent biography his grand-daughter described him as "the poster child for ADHD." He hit .340 for a career—and slept two hours a night. People like that need to stay busy.

Also remember that inmates lie. When you look at the sleep logs of people who complain that they can't sleep, the most common entry you find is "sound asleep."

Summary At bottom, we jail psychiatrists don't treat ADHD or sleep. The disabilities that ADHD causes are irrelevant to functioning in jail so they normally do not need treatment in jail. The symptoms of ADHD are easy to fake, so if we treated ADHD, inmates would feign symptoms to get ADHD drugs.

The only real exception to this is when an inmate is behaving in a way that causes CO's to talk to you. At that point you will want to do something (though not with stimulants).

Appendix IM
Inmate Management

Inmates cannot be trusted. They lie, cheat and steal. They have learned to do this from a young age. They have spent much of their time on this. Have some humility, doc. You can't have spent as much effort learning to penetrate all that as they have spent teaching themselves to perpetrate all that. For example, you spent your formative years in high school, college and medical school getting an education, while they were learning to lie, cheat and steal, getting their own kind of education. You will never be as good as they are at what they do.

What to do? You work in such a manner that when an inmate lies to you, he gets no benefit.

Specifically, this is what CO's will teach you in orientation classes or security briefings:

- Never leave an inmate in a room by himself. This also applies to inmate workers. In part, it is for their own safety. This way, they cannot be accused of stealing anything.

- Never trust an inmate. If you believe an inmate has made off with something, instantly tell a CO. The CO's will search the inmate.

- Never let an inmate near your stuff. Some of your stuff will disappear.

- We call inmate workers inmate workers because we do not call them 'trusties.' Calling someone a trustee implies that you trust him. We do not. You should not.

- You are there to do psychiatric business. That means diagnosing and treating mental illness. If the inmate wants to do anything more than that, direct him to go through normal channels.

- Never do an inmate a "favor." If you do, the inmate will later use that as a wedge for more favors (look up the fable about letting the camel put his nose in your tent). Eventually you can get in trouble for the favors you do for an inmate. The inmate will cheerfully betray you for even the smallest rewards. Don't do the first favor, and you will never do the illicit favor. Stick to business—your business.

- If an inmate even asks for paper, a pen or a pencil, the answer is "No. Ask through Inmate Services" or Program Services etc. Never give an inmate anything except the time of day.

Sometimes inmates seem to act normally, asking "social" questions. Inmates do not care about your life. They only ask because they are looking for a way to entice you, or threaten you to do their will. Say "I am here to ask questions, not to answer them" and "We are here to talk about you, not me."

If an inmate seems hostile or volatile, do not hesitate to call for a CO to stand in close attendance. If the inmate objects, so be it. Often an inmate wishes to isolate you, but not because they can actually do something. They want to isolate you to intimidate you, bully you to get their way.

Often inmates loudly demand drugs. They try to intimidate you into succumbing to their will. This works for them on the street; they are counting on it working for them now. Sometimes only sticking to your guns and calling for a CO (usually it requires both) will allow you to withstand a bully. Do it, though: the more you refuse to prescribe drugs, the easier refusing will be. As the months go on and inmates know they cannot expect drugs from you, the less of this explosivity there will be.

Never believe it when an inmate tells you that only some drug will "work." This is almost always a lie. Where it is not a lie—now is the time to explore nondrug medications.

Appendix ME
Medications

The following are medications and drugs that should prove interesting to psychiatrists. The brand name commonly associated with the chemical is in parentheses. It is commonly trademarked. As should be usual, your medication-ordering software should alert you to adverse interactions. The number of interactions has grown to such dimensions that no single person can keep track of them all. Only major or common interactions will be mentioned here.

There is no way a small appendix like this can tell you everything you need to know about these chemicals. As part of your knowledge base you should already know the important aspects of prescribing and monitoring these. Instead, this appendix strives to tell you the jail-specific issues you should know when considering these medicines and drugs.

Acamprosate (Campral) helps dependent people reduce their alcohol use.

Acetylcysteine - see N-acetylcysteine (NAC).

Agomelatine is used in some non-US countries as an antidepressant.

Allopregnanolone – see brexanolone.

Alprazolam (Xanax) is a benzodiazepine. Call it alcohol in a pill. In fact, alprazolam withdrawal can cause shakes, DT's, hallucinosis and seizures, just like alcohol withdrawal. Alprazolam can trigger an abstaining alcoholic to start drinking again. Inmates sometimes refer to this as the "felony pill" and the "amnesia pill" because they wake up the next day having committed a violent crime with no recollection of doing so. Like an active alcoholic, an alprazolam user will go through withdrawal and detox phases.

Amantadine (Symmetrel) is an old anti-flu agent that also has antiparkinsonian properties. When used for the latter purposes, it is mainly used for akathisia and akinesia. In combination, these side effects can be excruciating, causing the afflicted patient to want to get up and pace, yet be unable to do so. This has driven some patients to become suicidal. The effect of amantadine can be dramatic in some cases and ineffective in others. As a practical matter, a dose of 100mg BID is appropriate. There is generally no need to use the official maximum of 400mg per day.

Amisulpride is an 'atypical' antipsychotic that is sold in Europe but not in the US. It is known for hyperprolactinemia. Recently, it has found some use in paraphrenia at 100mg per day. This condition is also known as late onset schizo-phrenia, which is otherwise difficult to treat.

Amitriptyline (Elavil) is a TCA. It is a so-called tertiary amine—the terminal amine is fully substituted. The main use of this medication used to be as an antidepressant. Antidepressant doses usually ranged from 150 to 250mg HS, depending on the combined levels of amitriptyline and its psychoactive metabolite nortriptyline. These days, it is mainly used for its pain-reducing and soporific properties. For those uses, doses of 25-50mg HS are prescribed. This medication will destabilize someone with true bipolar disorder. It should be avoided in such cases. Like all TCA's, amitriptyline can be fatal in overdose. TCA's should not be used in a jail environment.

Amoxapine (Asendin) is a second-generation antidepressant. Amoxapine is a tetracyclic molecule related to loxapine. It came out when TCA's were on the market and was never very popular. Some psychiatrists think it is wonderful, however. Probably unavailable at your jail.

Amphetamine (Adderall) is a simulant, the original "speed." It is a medicine used to treat ADHD. It is also used to prolong wakefulness. Amphetamine differs from methylphenidate, because when it goes into synaptic vesicles, it displaces dopamine, norepinephrine, serotonin and other monoamines. Like methylphenidate, it increases intrasynaptic catecholamines by inhibiting their reuptake. Thus, amphetamine is a stronger stimulant than methylphenidate and will sometimes work when the latter will not. Amphetamine is not prescribed in jails.

Anti-anxiety agents – see anxiolytics.

Antipsychotics are used to combat psychosis, such as you find in schizophrenia, mania, toxicities and drug-induced psychoses. Antipsychotics are divided into first-generation and second-generation, often called 'typical' and 'atypical' antipsychotics. More recently, a third generation of antipsychotics has been emerging.

Anxiolytics are a class of medications that combat anxiety. Many medicines do this, including TCA's (especially amitriptyline and doxepin), antihistamines (especially hydroxyzine and diphenhydramine), benzodiazepines, buspirone, SNRI's, SSRI's and trazodone. TCA's are not used in jails because of their fatality in overdose situations. Antihistamines are comfort pills, "treating" those with no mental illness. They could be used outside of jails but not in jails. Benzodiazepines have been approved for anxiety, but benzodiazepines are 'alcohol in a pill' (see the specific listing). Buspirone is a true anxiolytic that has been approved for treatment of anxiety. Bupropion is usually thought of as a stimulant, but is an anxiolytic for some people; SNRI's are like SSRI's: they treat both anxiety and depression. Trazodone is an antidepressant used most often as a sleeping pill, precluding its use in jails.

Aripiprazole (Abilify) is very popular in the community. It is a second-generation antipsychotic with all of the baggage of those medicines. Yet because it has a reduced propensity to cause hyperprolactinemia and because it can be an adjunct for depression, it is used for a variety of purposes. In a state hospital, we found it not to be a very strong antipsychotic, but it had its uses. One aspect was that it comes in six formulations: tablet, dissolving tablet, liquid, acute IM, long-acting IM for monthly use and extra-long-acting IM for three-monthly use. This medication may not be on your jail's formulary (anticompetitive practices among generic drug manufacturers may keep the price high). But since it is not a drug, there are no contraindications to an inmate continuing to take the medication in jail.

An interesting potential adverse effect, especially likely in nonpsychotic individuals, is a heightened propensity for impulsive acts. Since it is a partial dopamine antagonist, it can in some circumstances act as a dopamine agonist. Since some antiparkinsonian medicines are dopamine agonists and those have been associated with impulsive acts, it is hardly surprising that aripiprazole might do the same. At the time of this writing, the extent of this effect is not fully known. But you should keep this in mind if you consider using this medication in a patient who is not psychotic.

Armodafanil (Nuvigil) is a derivative of modafanil. The effects are similar. It is not prescribed in jails.

Asenapine (Saphris) is one of the newer antipsychotics. This is the antipsychotic that is taken sublingually, presenting extra compliance issues, especially in a jail setting. This medication is probably not on your jail's formulary. But since it is not a drug, there are no contraindications to an inmate continuing to take the medication in jail. It does have potentially serious interactions with lisinopril. Check before prescribing.

Atypical antipsychotic is an unfortunate name for the second generation of antipsychotic medications. The name refers to the fact that these chemicals were designed not to produce EPS side effects; but they do! (Akathisia is a problem.) They just have fewer EPS side effects than the first generation of antipsychotics. "Atypical" antipsychotics target other receptors in addition to the dopamine receptors that the first generation of antipsychotics targeted.

Baclofen is an antispastic agent and muscle-relaxing agent. It is derived from GABA. It is included here because withdrawal from baclofen can resemble a BZD or alcohol withdrawal. It can worsen an alcohol or BZD withdrawal. So extra precautions against withdrawal should be taken when an inmate has been taking baclofen and it has been discontinued.

Barbiturates (multiple) are drugs. They are also fatal in overdose. Barbiturates are not used for any psychiatric purpose in a jail.

Benzodiazepines (Ativan, Dalmane, Halcion, Klonopin, Librium, Restoril, Serax, Valium, Xanax) might as well be referred to as alcohol in a pill. When someone uses them, she is liable to do things she would not do if she were clean (disinhibition). They impair her memory whether on an acute or a chronic basis. She can become dependent upon them to function—they allow her to feel she has coped with circumstances without her learning to do so. She can get strung out on them and come down with all the effects of an alcohol withdrawal: shakes, seizures, delirium tremens, and hallucinosis. Long term, benzodiazepines lead to an increased risk of dementia. These drugs should be used (if at all) on an emergent basis only, and then only briefly. See the No-PRN rule in Chapter 7 (page 168).

A better treatment for anxieties is usually to be found in psychology. There are psychological techniques that can help a person master her anxieties. But when her symptoms are covered up with benzodiazepines, she is unmotivated to pursue psychological treatments.

Benzodiazepines impair sleep architecture, so they are not a good choice as a routine treatment for sleep. As "comfort pills," benzodiazepines have no place in the routine treatment of mental disorders in jail settings. As addictive substances, they have no place in jails. Because there is a market for them, they have no place in jails. Avoid benzodiazepines.

Benztropine (Cogentin) is an anticholinergic antiparkinsonian agent used to counteract the EPS side effects of antipsychotics, especially first generation antipsychotics. It also has the benefit of lifting a patient's spirits. Benztropine has little utility in akinesia or akathisia, although it can be tried before other agents are tried. Although benztropine is usually thought to have less potential for abuse than other meds, I have seen it used to get a daily high, much like that of jimson weed. It can produce an anticholinergic toxicity, even when held to the maximum dose of 2mg TID; so care should be taken in prescribing it.

Beta Blockers are blood pressure pills that are used to treat essential tremor, akathisia and unwanted fearfulness. Since they are blood pressure pills, psychiatrists should not prescribe them in a jail.

Biperiden (Akineton) is an old anticholinergic. It used to be an unusual treatment for neuroleptic-induced pseudoparkinsonism. No longer used.

Bremelanotide (Vyleesi) An injectable medication for low libido. Libido? In jail?

Brexanolone (Zulresso) also known as allopregnanolone. Approved to treat post-partum depression. Before you get your hopes up, look this up to see how it interacts with GABA-A.

Brexpiprazole is a third generation antipsychotic. It has also been used as an adjunct in treating depression. It is new, so it will probably not be on your formulary.

Botulinum Toxin A (BTA) is best known for its applications in cosmetic work. However, it has shown some promise in depression and BPD. You will not be using this in jails.

Bupropion (Wellbutrin, Zyban) is an antidepressant that is used off-label to reduce the symptoms of ADHD. Controlled-release bupropion can be used to reduce smoking. There are two extended-release formulations, but the extended release property can be defeated by crushing it. When snorted, this can give the user an amphetamine-like high. That is why this medication is banned in some institutions and strictly controlled in others. The dose can range from 75 to 450mg per day, depending on release properties.

However—this is important—*the max dose of the immediate release form of bupropion is 150mg.*

When the dose is greater, the user risks seizures. In fact, this medicine was withdrawn from the market when it was first introduced until its relation to seizures could be explored. The highest dose of the CR form is 200mg at a time. The pill sizes of the XL form are 150mg, 300mg and 450mg, though the 450mg size is probably not available at your jail. Remember too that this chemical may be banned at your jail because of its history of abuse. Inmates may snort crazy amounts to get high; they risk seizures that way.

Bupropion often stimulates patients. Some cannot tolerate this effect. Yet there are others for whom bupropion calms their anxiety. This may be from its positive effects in ADHD. In any case, its use in jails is problematic.

Buspirone (Buspar) Aside from antidepressants, this is the sole treatment for anxiety allowed in a jail. Buspirone is not related to antidepressants, benzodiazepines or antihistamines. It is not habit-forming, and has few side effects, but it should not be used while or soon after someone has taken an MAOI. The doses range from 5 to 30mg BID. This medicine can surprise with its helpfulness across a broad variety of conditions, including ADHD. If it does not help her, an inmate should discontinue it.

Some jails do not allow buspirone. Inmates can crush and snort the tablets, thus abusing it. Doing this seems only to accelerate the onset of effects. It is not clear that inmates are potentially harming themselves (as with bupropion) when they crush and snort the tablet. As usual, more information is needed.

Cannabidiol (CBD) Approved by the FDA for treatment of two rare childhood-onset seizure disorders. No psychiatric indications.

Carbamazepine (Tegretol) is an anticonvulsant. There was early interest in this because it can help with manic episodes. In particular, it seemed to be helpful when used in combination with lithium. With the advent of divalproex, carbamazepine has been used a lot less in psychiatry, despite being weight-neutral, where valproate and divalproex can cause weight gain.

WARNING – The FDA has a warning that the risk of SJS/TEN in some Asian countries is estimated to be about 10 times higher than other populations. Thus, patients with ancestry in genetically at-risk populations should be screened for the presence of HLA-B*1502 prior to initiating treatment with carbamazepine. That broadly means that you should not initiate treatment in a person with Asian heritage. This can be a problem in some parts of the country. Please look up the latest guidance from the FDA.

Interestingly, carbamazepine seems to calm people down who were born as "crack babies," people who we now know have a diagnosis of ND-PAE. Carbamazepine seems help people in general who have a history of ND-PAE, IED or other forms of recurrent violence. Unfortunately, the other medication known to reduce violence—fluoxetine—can interact with carbamazepine, causing ataxia, among other issues. This is a reason to switch out one or the other of them. Oxcarbazepine might be a useful alternative.

Carbamazepine is useful in cases where the inmate has temporal lobe issues such as TLD. Neurologists usually prescribe lamotrigine for this condition, but that medicine is not safe to start in a jail environment. But carbamazepine may not be much safer (see above). An alternative is oxcarbazepine, which is normally given in 50% larger doses.

If you do start carbamazepine, start at the lowest possible dose—100mg BID—before going to 200mg BID, which seems to help some inmates. Do not further increase the dose until you get a blood level. Do not go above the therapeutic range of 4-12mg/L.

One advantage of carbamazepine is that it is weight-neutral; it does not cause obesity.

Carfentanil/carfentanyl (Wildnil) is an opiate, a synthetic analog of fentanyl and 10,000 times more potent than morphine. Not used by doctors in jails.

If an inmate overdoses on (presumably smuggled) opiates and more than one injector of naloxone is needed to bring him out of it, then you can conclude the inmate overdosed on carfentanyl or fentanyl, not heroin alone.

Cariprazine is a new antipsychotic. It has also been approved as an adjunct in treating depression. It is new, so it will probably not be on your formulary.

Carisoprodol (Soma) is a drug. It is a carbamate and is similar to barbiturates. Carbamates can be fatal in overdoses. Carisoprodol is not used for any psychiatric purposes in a jail.

Chlorpromazine (Thorazine) is the oldest antipsychotic. It is also an antihistamine, so it is sedating and anxiolytic. Before the common use of methylphenidate for ADHD, chlorpromazine was used to treat that. I have seen it misused in a jail setting, with chlorpromazine used to treat "depression" when in actuality what they were treating was ADHD symptoms and putting inmates to sleep. The problem with using chlorpromazine in this way is that like all first generation antipsychotics, it can cause tardive dyskinesia.

Inmates who appear to have developed their psychosis not from schizophrenia but from drug use, seem to do better taking a low-potency medication like chlorpromazine than they do with a high-potency antipsychotic. The problem is that many inmates, especially those with ADHD, want chlorpromazine not for its antipsychotic properties, but for the sedation it brings. They will fake being psychotic in order to get a pill that will damage them in the long run. Since a number of them shoot heroin of unknown provenance into their veins, often with shared needles, you can see that this poor judgment is not limited to psychotropic medications. So even if they don't care, you should. Chlorpromazine has no place in jail psychiatry.

Citalopram (Celexa) is a so-called SSRI. It is an antidepressant with anxiety-reducing properties. It seems to be the "cleanest" of the SSRI's, affecting other receptors less than it affects serotonin receptors. This is the classic medicine which treats an illness but does not "help" people without a psychiatric disorder. What is interesting is that this medicine sometimes seems to help people who have ADHD and who complain of depression. Their ADHD symptoms improve right along with their depressive symptoms.

One fly in the ointment of citalopram and its S-enantiomer escitalopram is that with moderately high doses there is a lengthened QTc interval. You cannot legally prescribe more than 40mg QD of citalopram or 20mg QD of escitalopram (there are some subgroups where the max is half that of normals). Those are stringent limitations; often an inmate seems to be almost there in his treatment. But it is better to switch from a medication that is helping, than to provoke a cardiac arrest.

Methadone also can prolong the QTc. It is contraindicated with citalopram.

Omeprazole can cause higher levels of citalopram. This is a medication commonly used with GERD, so you should note whether the inmate is taking this and reduce the citalopram.

Citalopram and escitalopram can cause a discontinuation syndrome if they are stopped suddenly, especially if they are discontinued from the maximum dose. This seems to be less of a problem when the inmate is switched to another SSRI. Sometimes the inmate himself has already stopped taking the medication. Then the order can be stopped without risking a discontinuation syndrome.

Citalopram should be a mainstay in your psychiatric armamentarium at jails.

Clomipramine (Anafranil) is a TCA. This medication was brought into the US on an orphan drug status to treat OCD, which it does very well. It has been used off-label to treat depression and anxiety. It is an outstanding treatment for anxiety and anxious depression, including otherwise refractory depression. Unfortunately, it can also cause seizures. Because it can act like a drug, it should not be used in jails. Because it is a TCA, it cannot be used in jails. If you use it outside jails, check EKG's.

Clonazepam (Klonopin) is a BZD. It was brought to market as an anticonvulsant (Clonopin, as it was then called, referenced the tonic-clonic actions of grand mal seizures) but is now most used as an anxiolytic. Some doctors believe it is a superior anxiolytic to alprazolam, since it has a much longer half-life. But it is still a benzodiazepine. Do not use it.

Clonidine (Catapress) is a medication that inhibits the release of epinephrine by interacting with receptors on the cells that release epinephrine. It was initially marketed as a blood pressure pill, and a sublingual dose of clonidine can emergently reduce critically high blood pressure. It can be used to blunt the effects of withdrawal from a number of substances, especially opiates. Apparently, it can also be used to treat RLS. Side effects of clonidine include low blood pressure, dry mouth and lethargy.

For psychiatry, clonidine is a versatile tool. Clonidine can be used to treat various symptoms of ADHD, tics (especially those found in Tourette's disorder) and TD. It can be used emergently to reduce nonpsychotic distress. Clonidine can be used as a drug to treat anxiety; but for anxiety it is a drug, not a medicine.

Clonidine has not proven to be successful at suppressing the nightmares of PTSD. Although some doctors use it for this, the effects are more likely those of a nighttime anxiolytic or a nighttime reduction of ADHD symptoms.

When you have access to blood pressure readings of inmates, you should not start clonidine if the systolic is below 110mm Hg. When you prescribe it, you should pay attention to any lightheadedness. Inmates should be warned that clonidine can reduce blood pressure. If they ever feel lightheaded at all they should sit right down. They should not try to fight the medicine; the medicine will win.

For the most part, I no longer prescribe clonidine. It is too much a drug, and it allows an inmate to escape coping with her problems. Since it is an antihypertensive, only a medical specialist should prescribe clonidine.

Clozapine (Clozaril) is an antipsychotic—the first "atypical," in that it produces EPS side effects less often than other first-generation antipsychotics. The trouble with clozapine, is that it is potentially fatal through neutropenia and agranulo-cytosis. Why would the patient and the patient's doctors take such risks? This medication is the last resort. It will treat cases of psychosis that are refractory to all other treatments. You need to register with clozapinerems.com to use this medication.

If an inmate comes in taking clozapine, you should continue it to prevent a clozapine with-drawal syndrome. If you do not have much exper-ience with this medication, reach out to a colleague who does. Usually the local state hospit-al will have prescribers who are familiar with managing patients who take this medication. Try to arrange for your own direct access to the lab doing the CBC, so that you can track the WBC and ANC (absolute neutrophil count) quickly. There are online resources to give you guidelines for treating with this dangerous medication.

Try never to start someone on clozapine. From clinical experience, it seems that in cases where clozapine has been used before it becomes the last resort, after clozapine nothing else will work. So you must be sure that nothing less potentially fatal will work before you try cloza-pine; hence, don't start this in a jail. More than other second-generation antipsychotics, cloza-pine causes obesity, dyslipidemia and diabetes mellitus.

Patients with intellectual disability may get treated with antipsychotics to control their behav-ior. When this treatment fails, the providers may escalate their chemical assault. Be sure you are treating psychosis when you continue clozapine.

Cyclobenzaprine (Flexeril) It may seem odd to you that a nonpsychiatric drug is included here. Back in the 1980's I had a patient whose depression went away when he took cyclobenzaprine. I investigated. Looking at a picture of the molecule in the PDR, it was clear that it looked like a TCA. Investigating further, I called the manufacturer (you reached real people on the phone in those days). I spoke with one of the developers. He said that they had derived this medication from amitriptyline. Unfortunately, it was successful only 30% of the time, so they found another market for the chemical, even giving it a non-TCA generic name.

The reason cyclobenzaprine is included here is that even with a non-TCA name, it still acts like a TCA. If a person is taking cyclobenzaprine, he should not be given an MAOI. Proceed carefully if you have to start a TCA; and follow all the precautions you would if you were prescribing a medication in conjunction with a TCA. There is no reason for a psychiatrist to prescribe this in a jail.

Cyproheptadine (Periactin) is an anti–histamine and it is used for medical—not psychiatric—purposes in a jail. It is also a drug, so there are further reasons not to use it in jail. However, cyproheptadine has been used off-label to treat serotonin syndrome, PTSD nightmares, and SSRI-induced sexual dysfunction. But without an official psychiatric indication, there is no reason for a psychiatrist to prescribe this in a jail setting.

D-cycloserine (Seromycin) is an antibiotic used to treat TB. There is some evidence that it may be useful in a number of psychiatric conditions. The psychiatric uses are experimental, so you should not use it in a jail.

Desipramine (Norpramin) is a TCA. Because it is generally non-sedating, it is not usually a drug. One time in a jail I broke my no-TCA rule, because an inmate was chronically very agitated. He seemed to calm down with this treatment. But we discovered later that he liked the pill, and it was a drug for him. So he hoarded it and took an overdose trying to get a real "high." We were lucky the OD did not kill him. Since then, we have not deviated from our no-TCA rule.

This medication will destabilize someone with true bipolar disorder. It should be avoided in such cases. Desipramine should not be used in a jail environment.

Desvenlafaxine (Pristiq) is an active metabolite of venlafaxine. Like venlafaxine, it is an SNRI. Also like venlafaxine, it can produce a discontinuation syndrome, complete with the sensation of electric shocks in the brain. This will destabilize someone with true bipolar disorder. It should be avoided in such cases.

Deutetrabenazine (Austedo) has been approved to treat tardive dyskinesia and Huntington's Disease chorea.

Dexmethylphenidate (Focalin) is an active stereoisomer of methylphenidate. It is similar to its parent compound.

Dextroamphetamine (Dexedrine) is an

active stereoisomer of amphetamine. It is similar to its parent compound.

Dextromethorphan (Nuedexta) can be given in combination with quinidine, which inhibits its metabolism and causes the dextromethorphan level to rise more than 20-fold. This combination seems to greatly reduce agitation in delirious demented patients. It should not be needed in jails, but recall that antipsychotics are usually prescribed in these cases, and antipsychotics are deadly in dementia. Although the DXM by itself is generic, OTC and cheap, the combination is not. If you have a delirious demented person in your jail, get him to a physical hospital quickly.

I did run into a case of pseudobulbar palsy in a jail. The inmate thought his problem was psychiatric and did not link it to his TBI. Clearly, his insight and judgment were impaired along with his affect.

Diphenhydramine (Benadryl) is an antihistamine with some sedating properties. As an antihistamine, it can bring blessed relief to itching within an hour after taking it PO. That use is medical, not psychiatric, however. Psychiatrically, diphenhydramine can be used as an alternative to benztropine. Unfortunately, monopolistic behavior by some generic pharmaceutical manufacturers will sometimes leave only one producer of a particular medication. In such a case, the manufacturer may jack the price of its medication sky high. Perhaps fortunately, the utility of diphenhydramine means that the market for it will always remain competitive, and the price will be relatively low. If such considerations lead you to prescribing this, just remember that this is a desirable drug. Some inmates seek it, chasing its sleep-inducing properties (unfortunately for them, this property fades with time). For most inmates, then, diphenhydramine is a drug. Where such drugs are prescribed, a market will grow up in your jail for this substance.

Disulfiram (Antabuse) reduces alcohol consumption by producing nausea and other unpleasant effects. Introduced in 1950, for a long time it was all we had.

Divalproex (Depakote) is an anticonvulsant that was discovered to be useful in bipolar disorder. Thus it may be for medical or psych. Divalproex is a derivative of valproic acid (VPA). Divalproex is converted to VPA by the liver. VPA causes GI disturbance in 20% of patients. Divalproex reduces that to 10%. Divalproex is usually given BID. If the ER form is available to you and you prescribe it, the medicine should be given once a day.

In some places, divalproex is commonly used in schizophrenia. The practice probably got started because psychiatrists were trying to prevent people with bipolar schizoaffective disorder from becoming manic. But there are no RCT's to support this practice; divalproex has not been found to improve functioning in schizophrenia. When doctors use it in schizophrenia, they are either treating genuine bipolar schizoaffective disorder or they are tacitly admitting that they don't know what they are treating.

Divalproex sometimes is used to calm people down during their rehabilitation from drugs. It may cushion events and inhibit the emotional excursions of the detoxed individual.

Divalproex occasionally helps people with ND-PAE. But normally it is not too helpful for this or for TLD. Carbamazepine is generally preferable for those disorders. But also generally, if an inmate does better taking divalproex, there is no reason not to continue it.

When you have someone who has had emotional disturbances from childhood, they almost certainly do not have real bipolar disorder. They probably have DMDD, but you should ask about adverse childhood events. More importantly, you should not blindly continue divalproex in an inmate on the theory that the treating psychiatrist "must know what he is doing." Probably he does not. Don't treat someone with divalproex unless he or she truly has bipolar disorder, or some other condition known to respond to it.

You should already know how to prescribe and manage divalproex. A few caveats: this medicine can produce weight gain, sometimes-massive weight gain. Monitor your patients for this. Divalproex causes birth defects in pregnancy and when those children grow older they have characteristic features and disabilities. It should not normally be used in pregnancy. Divalproex is a cruel med to give to children: it shortens their stature. Divalproex and valproic acid can also cause polycystic ovary syndrome (PCOS) and because of its known birth defects, it is contraindicated in women of childbearing age. Finally, divalproex and VPA can cause elevation of liver enzymes. This can be monitored by drawing periodic LFT's.

Donepezil (Aricept) is used to treat Alzheimer's Disease. It succeeds only mildly.   See discussion under memantine.

Doxepin (Sinequan) is a TCA and cannot be used in jails. Even when it is given in a liquid form, inmates can soak a tissue with the liquid and either store it up for themselves (dangerous) or hand it off to another inmate who has no compunctions about eating used tissue. This is also dangerous, with an additional yuck factor; but after all, they do share needles, so they have no problem with sharing oral products.

Doxepin is an excellent anxiolytic antidepressant. It can help even someone with ADHD find sleep, so not only is it sold as an antidepressant, there is a very-low-dose form available to treat insomnia. Outside jail, former inmates often can benefit from this druglike medicine. But it should not be used in jail.

This medication will destabilize someone with true bipolar disorder. It should be avoided in such cases.

Side effects tend to be anticholinergic. Large doses can kill.

Duloxetine (Cymbalta) is an SNRI. It was developed as an antidepressant, but it also may be prescribed for pain, especially neuropathic pain. Do ask the inmate whether she was taking this for pain or psych. If she was taking this for pain, the medical specialist must order it. For psychiatry, the dose ranges from 30 to 120mg QAM, though you may see it given BID. It is not normally soporific, so use in jail is OK, depending on formulary considerations. Some patients can experience a discontinuation syndrome if it is stopped suddenly, especially with large doses. The syndrome is harmless, though uncomfortable. Your jail may or may not have this on its formulary. If so, feel free to use it.

Ecstasy (MDMA) In Phase III trials for treatment-resistant PTSD. See MDMA.

Escitalopram (Lexapro) is an SSRI. It is an active stereoisomer of citalopram (Celexa). Some people can tolerate escitalopram who cannot tolerate racemic citalopram. In RCT's it helps about 3% more people than citalopram.

One fly in the ointment of citalopram and its S-enantiomer escitalopram is that with moderately high doses there is a lengthened QTc interval. You cannot legally prescribe more than 40mg QD of citalopram or 20mg QD of escitalopram (there are some subgroups where the max is half that of normals). Those are stringent limitations; often an inmate seems to be almost there in his treatment. But it is better to switch from a medication that is helping than to provoke a cardiac arrest.

Methadone also can prolong the QTc. It is contraindicated with escitalopram.

Omeprazole can cause higher levels of citalo-pram (and presumably escitalopram). This is a medication commonly used with GERD so you should note whether the inmate is taking this or not. Escitalopram and citalopram can cause a discontinuation syndrome if they are stopped suddenly. Look at the entry on citalopram for details.

Esketamine (Spravato) is a nasal drug approved by the FDA for TRD. Esketamine is the S-enantiomer of ketamine, which is a legal anes-thetic that has been used to get high. Recent studies have found that pretreating with naltrex-one blocks the antidepressant effect of ketamine, so it may be an opioid. There are other controversies, as well.

An esketamine user is supposed to use the esketamine nasal spray while supervised by a provider in a certified doctor's office. A user is not allowed to take the drug home. Further, users have to be monitored by a healthcare provider for at least 2 hours after getting the drug.

You can see that you are not likely to be using this drug soon in a jail setting.

Eszopiclone (Lunesta) is a sleeping pill, and thus not appropriate for jails.

Ezogabine (Potiga in the US) (the generic name is retigabine outside the US) is an anticon-vulsant which may have antidepressant propert-ies. It was withdrawn from the US market due to concerns over side effects.

Fentanyl (Durogesic or Duragesic patches) is an opiate analog, 50-100 times more potent than morphine. If more than one injection of naloxone is needed in an overdose, the person has used fentanyl or carfentanyl, not just heroin.

First-Generation Antipsychotic — also called a neuroleptic or a "typical" antipsychotic. These medicines are known for akathisia, akinesia and 'extra-pyramidal system' side effects like dystonia and pseudoparkinsonism. Famously, high-potency first-generation antipsychotics are associated with tardive dyskinesia. They are considered neurotoxic today.

Flibanserin (Addyi) is a medication for low libido. Libido? Really? In jail?

Flumazenil competitively inhibits benzodiazepines. It is used to rescue people who are suffering from an overdose of benzodiazepines. Unfortunately, this medication can also cause seizures and agitation. Quite a few benzodiazepines have longer half-lives than flumazenil, so repeated administration may be needed to prevent recurrence of overdose symptoms when the flumazenil wears off.

Although you would be hard pressed to find flumazenil in most jails, stats tell us that benzodiazepine abuse is growing rapidly. Expect jails to be forced to respond.

Fluoxetine (Prozac) is the original SSRI: it was first approved at the end of 1987. It has been used successfully in the treatment of depression, anxiety, anger, rage, obsessions, compulsions, bulimia, anorexia, trichotillomania, PMD, PMS and post-stroke violence. Dosage rages from

10mg QAM (post-stroke) to 20mg QAM (depression) to 80mg (OCD; 40mg BID).

This medicine is usually given in the morning, because it can keep recipients awake if given at night. Yet when given in the morning it can improve sleep in depressed subjects at night. It can produce nausea, which will fade. Sexual and urinary effects do not fade and are reasons to stop the med or switch.

Fluoxetine is known for its ability to reduce anger; yet it can provoke anger and akathisia. Some people do well with it; some people do poorly with it. All you can do is try it, with the instruction that the inmate should stop taking the medicine if it makes him feel worse.

Unfortunately, the other medication known to reduce violence—carbamazepine—can interact with fluoxetine, causing ataxia, among other issues. This is a reason to swap out one or the other of them.

Fluphenazine (Prolixin) is a neuroleptic. Of all of the first-generation antipsychotics it was the most potent, having about 70 times as much antipsychotic power as chlorpromazine. The antipsychotic dose is about 5mg per day. Like all first generation antipsychotics, fluphenazine can cause akathisia, akinesia, dystonia and pseudo-parkinsonism—the EPS litany. It is usually given with benztropine or diphenhydramine. Fluphenazine is often switched with haloperidol, since they are both similarly potent and they produce essentially the same side effects. For inmates who are taking haloperidol or fluphenazine, you should comment on their TD status. A convenient place to do this is in the mental status examination (MSE).

As an interesting side note, there seems to be no ceiling on the effect of fluphenazine. It can be given in strikingly large doses to shut psychoses down. These days, it is best not to exceed the approved maximum of 40mg per day.

Another interesting issue is cost. As the demand for these older meds has fallen, the generic med makers seem to have consolidated what they make. So instead of two or more companies competing for your company's business, one company will make drug A, one will make drug B, etc. Your company may change what meds are available on your formulary based on shifting costs.

Just before the second generation of antipsychotics were released, there was a movement to use smaller doses of high-potency antipsychotics. Doctors were finding better success in some cases by reducing doses to 1-2mg instead of increasing to 20mg. The advent of second-generation antipsychotics put an end to this broad informal experiment by psychiatrists, but it is something to keep in mind. It is especially important, because studies have shown that patients are just as happy with first-generation antipsychotics as with second-generation medications. It would behoove practitioners to keep the doses of first-generation meds as low as possible to avoid tardive dyskinesia.

Fluphenazine Decanoate (Prolixin-D) is a depot formulation. The active medication is bound to decanoic acid in an ester form, and released over the next few weeks as the medicine dissociates from the fatty acid. In the vial, the fluphenazine is present in equilibrium of free and bound fluphenazine. Usually this is not important, but in a few cases people need an anticholinergic when they get their antipsychotic-decanoate injections. Decanoate injections are given because you can give an older antipsychotic with far fewer unpleasant side effects than with oral medication.

Calculate the monthly dose of a decanoate by multiplying the daily dose by ten. For fluphenazine-decanoate the monthly dose is spread out over four weeks with half given every two weeks.

Fluphenazine decanoate is available in 25mg (1 mL) vials. It is usually given in 25mg injections every two weeks (5mg PO per day PO x 10 = 50mg decanoate IM across four weeks, so 25mg every 2 weeks). The maximum dose is actually the number of ml that can be injected in the same syringe. That used to be 3ml. Now the maximum dose is more often 2ml.

Fluvoxamine (Luvox) is An SSRI. Its primary use is for OCD, because it can cause a variety of side effects. As an SSRI, it can be used to treat depression and anxiety. Some practitioners have used it to treat panic disorder and PTSD. The controlled release (CR) form has been approved to treat social phobia (social anxiety disorder). Probably, clomipramine is a better treatment for

OCD. Fluvoxamine is not on the formulary of most jails.

Gabapentin (Neurontin) is an anticonvulsant. It also is used to reduce pain, especially neuropathic pain. It is NOT a mood-stabilizer like divalproex. There are NO approved psychiatric uses. You may think that gabapentin has legitimate purposes, but that is not accurate. It is targeted at the GABA receptors, just like the benzodiazepines; but it does not strongly bind to any of them. While the mechanism of what gabapentin does is still not known, the actions of this drug are known. It will calm people down.

It will calm anyone down. That makes gabapentin a drug. Some people abuse this drug and get addicted to it. It should not be used in jails. No, your legitimate bipolar patients will not develop mania without their gabapentin, but your borderline and drug-dependent inmates will clamor for their missing drug. They can do without it. Psychiatrists sometimes prescribe gabapentin for anxiety, thinking to evade the prohibition against benzodiazepines. Don't do it.

New information on gabapentin. NJ practitioners received the following email: "Effective May 7, 2018, the New Jersey Division of Consumer Affairs . . . require New Jersey licensed pharmacies and registered out-of-State pharmacies to electronically transmit information to the Division about prescriptions dispensed for gabapentin. The recognition of gabapentin as a "drug of concern" stems from national prescription and overdose data. New Jersey is joining a growing list of states who have already begun to monitor gabapentin use, including those that have scheduled the medication at the state level.

"Studies have shown that gabapentin prescribing in the United States has increased 49% over the past five years resulting in 64 million prescription dispensations in 2016. Additionally, the prevalence of gabapentin abuse in the general population is only 1.2%, but increases to a staggering 15% - 22% amongst opioid users; likely a direct result of the potentiating effects caused by combination therapy. In New Jersey, over the past two years, the presence of gabapentin in post-mortem toxicology reports increased by more than 1,000% overall and by more than 3,000% in the opioid-use subgroup."

Galantamine is used to treat Alzheimer's Disease. See discussion under Memantine.

Guanfacine (Tenex) Like clonidine, this medication inhibits the release of epinephrine by interacting with receptors on the cells that release epinephrine. It was initially marketed as a blood pressure pill. It is mildly successful at this, but its main use is in the treatment of ADHD, especially the hyperactivity component. According to a recent study, guanfacine may improve executive functioning in ADHD; time will tell, but ADHD *per se* is not something we treat in an adult jail. Like clonidine, guanfacine may or may not be helpful in reducing the nightmares of PTSD. It has been successful in treating tics associated with ADHD but its use with other forms of tic is uncertain. Guanfacine can be used to treat anxiety, but for anxiety it is a drug, not a medicine. So guanfacine has no place in the psychiatric armamentarium of an adult jail.

Haloperidol (Haldol) is a neuroleptic. Of all of the first generation of antipsychotics it was the second most potent, having about 60 times as much antipsychotic power as chlorpromazine. The antipsychotic dose is about 5mg per day. Like all first-generation antipsychotics, haloperidol can cause akathisia, akinesia, dystonia and pseudoparkinsonism—the whole EPS litany. It is usually given with benztropine or diphenhydramine. Haloperidol is often switched with fluphenazine, since they are both similarly potent and they produce essentially the same side effects. For inmates who are taking haloperidol or fluphenazine, you should comment on their TD status. A convenient place to do this is in the mental status examination (MSE).

As an interesting side note, there seems to be a ceiling on the effect of haloperidol. It seems that for the typical patient, when you use above 20-30mg per day, you will get no stronger effect than if you stay at 20-30mg per day. There are a few exceptions.

Another interesting issue is cost. As the demand for these older meds has fallen, the generic drug makers seem to have consolidated what they make. So instead of two or more companies competing for your company's business one company will make medicine X, one will make medicine Y, etc. Your company may change what meds are available on your formulary based on shifting costs.

Just before the second generation of antipsychotics was released, there was a movement to use smaller doses of high-potency antipsychotics. Doctors were finding better success in some cases by reducing doses to 1-2mg instead of increasing to 20mg. The advent of second-generation antipsychotics put an end to this informal experiment by psychiatrists, but it is something to keep in mind. It is especially important, because studies have shown that patients are just as happy with first-generation antipsychotics as with second-generation medications. It would behoove practitioners to keep the doses of first-generation meds as low as possible to avoid tardive dyskinesia.

Haloperidol Decanoate (Haldol Dec) This is a depot formulation. The active medication is bound to decanoic acid in an ester form and released over the next few weeks as the medicine dissociates from the fatty acid. In the vial, the haloperidol is present in equilibrium of free and bound haloperidol. Usually this is not important, but in a few cases people need an anticholinergic when they get their antipsychotic-decanoate injections. Decanoate injections are given because you can give an older antipsychotic with far fewer unpleasant side effects than with oral medication.

Calculate the monthly dose of a decanoate by multiplying the daily dose by ten. For haloperidol decanoate, this is the number of mg given in monthly injections. Haloperidol decanoate is available as 50mg/ml and 100mg/ml. It is usually given in 50mg injections every four weeks (5mg PO per day oral x 10 = 50mg decanoate IM every month). The maximum dose is actually the number of ml that can be injected in the same syringe. The maximum dose used to be 3ml. Now the maximum dose is more often 2ml.

Heroin (generic) is an opiate with no psychiatric indications. It is a drug.

Hydroxyzine (Atarax, Vistaril) is an antihistamine. It can be used by the medical specialist as an antihistamine. People without mental illness can feel calmer or sleepy when they take it, so it is also a drug. Some doctors tout its abilities as an anxiolytic. It is not a benzodiazepine, so it is not habit-forming, they say. But when I was a student I recall that we gave our post-op patients hydroxyzine to reduce their need for opiates. Those patients were not mentally ill.

Hydroxyzine is a comfort pill. As a side note, I will observe that doctors were still trying to reduce the use of opiates in those days, trying to avoid producing iatrogenic opiate addicts. This was before the days of pain scales etc.

At bottom, prescribing this chemical is like prescribing a benzodiazepine, marijuana or even alcohol for a situational issue. If the inmate does not learn that he can survive a stressor like incarceration without dying or going insane, he will never be able to face a crisis without some kind of chemical help. You are saying you do not think the inmate can handle his life. You think he needs the drugs that doctors prescribe. You make him dependent on the medical profession.

In the end, prescribing hydroxyzine makes you little better than the corner drug dealer, only more inconvenient. It should not be prescribed by psychiatric practitioners in a jail setting.

Iloperidone (Fanapt) is a second-generation antipsychotic. This medication is probably not on your jail's formulary. But since it is not a drug, there are no contraindications to an inmate continuing to take the medication in jail.

Imipramine (Tofranil) is a TCA, and will destabilize someone with true bipolar disorder. It should be avoided in such cases. It can be fatal in overdose. TCA's like imipramine should not be used in a jail environment.

Kava (kava-kava) is a drug. It affects most people who imbibe it, and not just those with psychiatric disturbances. It has no place in a jail practice.

Ketamine This is a general anesthetic, the original "horse tranquilizer." It has actions at the NMDA receptor and other receptors. When used IV it has shown some promise as an antidepressant. It is also a "recreational drug." In a recent pilot study, it was seen to act faster than traditional calming agents in an ER. Also: recent studies have found that pretreating with naltrexone blocks the antidepressant effect. Does it work because it is an opioid?

Kratom is a drug with opiate properties. It

should not be used in a jail, even for opiate withdrawal.

Lamotrigine (Lamictal) Note: Lamotrigine can cause *Stevens-Johnson Syndrome* if it is started abruptly or increased rapidly. SJS is a potentially fatal illness. When an inmate comes in taking lamotrigine, ask her when she last took the med. If more than 4 days have passed she must NOT receive it. Even if it was ordered within the 4-day time frame, if she does not get the med within 4 days, STOP THE MEDICATION.

Lamotrigine is an anticonvulsant. It may be used for generalized seizures, for epilepsy, focal seizures, primary and secondary tonic-clonic seizures, seizures associated with Lennox-Gastaut syndrome, temporal lobe seizures or for temporal-limbic dysfunction.

Lamotrigine can treat the depression of true bipolar disorder. But because of SJS, it can be a tricky medication to use in jails. Start it only as a last resort in a jail, when you are sure that the inmate has a bipolar disorder, she is depressed and nothing else works. Also, it may not be on your formulary. NB – a recent study showed that, while it had promising indicators, lamotrigine is not helpful in BPD. Lamotrigine can also induce porphyria. Be careful with it.

Lisdexamfetamine (Vyvanse) is a pro-drug that is converted to amphetamine when it is metabolized in the liver. It is used to treat ADHD. Users report that it has a smoother onset than other stimulants, and lasts longer. Because this is a stimulant, it has not been used in jails.

Lithium (generic) is a medication that was introduced for the management of genuine bipolar disorder, also called 'bipolar type I' and 'manic-depressive illness.' The uses of lithium are still being explored. It seems to be more helpful in mania than depression, yet people who take it commit suicide less often than those who do not. People who take lithium can appear relaxed and even lackadaisical: back in the 1980's, when lithium was used more frequently, family practitioners could often tell who was taking it from their patient's demeanor. Lithium may take two weeks to work. Make sure you do not overtreat with antipsychotics while waiting for the lithium effect to kick in.

The side effects of lithium can include a tremor that looks like essential tremor, and like essential tremor it can be treated with propranolol. Lithium can also cause polyuria. The treatment for lithium-induced polyuria can include amiloride (a diuretic) but more realistically for a jail environment, just stop the lithium. Lithium can cause diarrhea. As levels increase, people can experience stupor, coma and death. Long-term effects of lithium can include hypothyroidism. Lithium must generally be given carefully in a patient who is receiving diuretics, but lisinopril in particular increases the side effects of lithium through unknown mechanisms.

Lithium seems to have at least two dosage ranges, one for therapeutic effects, and one for side effects. The two ranges appear to occur independently in different people. Some people are helped by low doses of lithium, where they do not experience many if any side effects. Other people cannot reach therapeutic levels without meeting side effects first, precluding their treatment with lithium.

Lithium not only helps to stabilize bipolar disorder; it can in low doses calm people who have ADHD. For people with ADHD, 300mg BID to TID helps them, and they run a level of 0.5 mmol/L or less—subtherapeutic for bipolar disorder; but more than that does not help them further, so you can ignore the blood level.

In a jail setting, undertreating with lithium is far safer than trying to reach a level of 1.0. In addition to the many side effects inmates will report, if their fluid intake is restricted, they may have an elevation of their lithium blood level. A low blood level will keep your inmate (and you) out of trouble.

In preparation for lithium therapy and managing lithium therapy, you should follow the latest professional guidelines. Since the most common reason that psychiatrists are sued is failure to monitor lithium treatment, monitor the drug levels, the kidney functions, the thyroid functioning and anything else that is recommended.

Lofexidine (Lucemyra) is a medicine first marketed for blood pressure control. It has now been approved for blunting the symptoms of opiate withdrawal.

Lorazepam (Ativan) is a benzodiazepine. The IM form can be used to treat acute episodes of psychotic agitation. But be sure it is agitation you are treating. For example, an inmate with an alleged history of psychosis threw an almighty fit one night and the nurse persuaded me to order a lorazepam injection. A couple of days later, the inmate became agitated again. She told the nurse that at the state hospital they had ordered a PRN when she became agitated. The nurse dutifully reported this (you have no better coadjutor than a good nurse) so this time I instructed the nurse to tell the inmate there would be no PRN. When I was done with my interview, I came over to where the inmate was housed. She was quiet and calm. She had not needed the PRN after all. This confirmed what I had seen at the state hospital: patients would stage episodes of 'agitation' to get a shot of lorazepam. Enough said.

Lorazepam appears to have unique properties in treating **catatonia**. Other benzodiazepines do not help this condition. Generally, if inmates require treatment for catatonia, then they belong in hospitals, not jails. Generally, do not prescribe lorazepam or any other benzodiazepine in jail.

Loxapine (Loxitane) is a first-generation antipsychotic that arguably behaved like a second-generation antipsychotic. Chemically, it is similar to clozapine. Loxapine does not cause agranulocytosis, nor the metabolic syndrome. It may be metabolized to amoxapine, an antidepressant. Loxapine is generic, so it has a possibility of being on a jail's formulary.

Major Tranquilizer This is an old term. These are usually antipsychotics. First-generation antipsychotic were called this.

MDMA (ecstasy; Molly) 3,4-Methylenedioxy-methamphetamine, a drug of abuse. Although this drug is now is Phase III trials for treating PTSD, it may not be allowed in jails. And even if it is, there will likely be stringent requirements for prior attempts at treatment for outside use. Any inmate who comes to you for MDMA should be in documented active treatment with a psychiatric physician, APN or PA to be considered at all. We should expect people lying to us to get this drug.

Melatonin is a hormone that helps to regulate diurnal rhythms in mammalian species. Because it is not standardized by the FDA, it is not provided in hospitals, jails, etc. Back in the early 1990's, when one could obtain pharmaceutical-grade melatonin, I once used it to regularize sleep in a patient with post-cardiotomy delirium, and cleared up her delirium. Yes, it was a study with an N of one, but it is interesting nonetheless. A related medication is ramelteon.

Memantine is used to treat Alzheimer's Disease. There is some controversy over whether a psychiatrist or a general medical doctor should prescribe this, since Alzheimer's is not strictly speaking a psychiatric disorder; yet this disease can affect behavior.

Methamphetamine (Desoxyn) Also known as "meth," this is a stimulant related to amphetamine (see). It is not prescribed in jails.

Methadone is a legal drug used to maintain opiate addicts so they can ostensibly lead law-abiding lives. The addicts typically must attend a clinic every day to get their drug. Unfortunately, the testimony of addicts indicates they often sell methadone on the street to generate funds, often for more desirable drugs. And despite what you are told, addicts can get high from heroin while taking methadone. You should keep in mind that methadone can prolong the QTc. This is a health risk by itself, and it is a contraindication for using citalopram concurrently.

Methylfolate (Deplin) is a methylated form of folic acid. According to a current theory, the methylated variety allows an activated form of folic acid to be present in individuals who have a reduced folic acid metabolism. Currently, it is marketed as an adjunct to antidepressant treatment. Supposedly, this should help most people who are depressed and overweight, especially those who have had adverse childhood experiences (ACE's). This may or may not make its way into jails in the future. Certainly it fits the population jail psychiatrists most often see.

Methylphenidate (Ritalin; controlled release: Concerta) A simulant, it is a medicine used to treat ADHD. It is also used to prolong wakefulness. Methylphenidate differs from amphetamine in that it does not displace monoamines from synaptic vesicles. Like amphetamine, it increases intrasynaptic norepinephrine and other monoamines by inhibiting their reuptake. Thus, methylphenidate is not as thoroughgoing a stimulant as amphetamine, and will sometimes not work when the latter will; but amphetamine is too strong for some people, so methylphenidate is used. Methylphenidate is short-acting and often requires multiple dosing to be effective across the day; hence the existence of controlled-release formulations. As a short-acting med, it can be used to initiate sleep in people with ADHD. Methylphenidate is not prescribed in adult jails.

Minor Tranquilizers An old term. These are usually anxiolytics, especially benzodiazepines, but the term might include barbiturates.

Mirtazapine (Remeron, "Ramrod") is an antidepressant—at doses of 30mg and up. Bio-chemical studies show effects on the serotonin system. As the dosage is increased, it has an ever-greater effect on the adrenergic system. So a dose of 7.5-15mg will produce drowsiness in most people, even if they do not have a mental illness. That means that mirtazapine is a drug in doses under 30mg. Mirtazapine is also associated with weight gain. Some studies indicate that an overdose can be problematic, even fatal.

This medication will destabilize someone with true bipolar disorder. Mirtazapine should be avoided in such cases. Mirtazapine in general should not be used in a jail environment.

Modafanil (Provigil) helps people stay awake. It is not used in jails.

Molindone (Moban) was a first-generation antipsychotic, allegedly producing less weight gain than other antipsychotics.

Morphine (generic) an old opiate.

N-acetylcysteine (NAC) is still used to thin the mucous of people with cystic fibrosis and to counteract acetaminophen overdose. It has been gaining currency as an adjunct in the treatment of depression and other psychiatric disorders. You may run into this, but it is hard to imagine taxpayers supporting an unproven therapy.

Nabilone (Cesamet) mimics THC, the active component of marijuana. This has been used off-label to "treat" nightmares.

Naloxone (Narcan) blocks the effects of opiates.

Naltrexone (ReVia and Vivitrol) is included here because it is possible that a psychiatrist might be tasked with starting it. Naltrexone is a mild opiate agonist for opiates and a major antagonist. Clinically, it tends to reduce a dependent person's craving, while blocking the "high" gotten from the substance. It was first approved to treat alcoholism, then opiate dependence.

Naltrexone is available as a pill, a three-monthly pellet, and a monthly injection (men have been known to cut the pellet out). It does not cause nausea when the subject uses his substance.

Nefazodone (Serzone) is an antidepressant that is mostly not used because of a potential to cause hepatotoxicity. It also causes drowsiness in most people who take it even if they do not have a mental illness. That means that nefazodone is a drug and should not be used in a jail.

Neuroleptics a name for first-generation

antipsychotics.

Nortriptyline (Aventyl, Pamelor) is a tricyclic antidepressant, a secondary amine derivative of amitriptyline. Both drugs are active antidepressants. When managing depression outside the jail with nortriptyline, measure nortriptyline levels.

Like many TCA's, nortriptyline has been used by nonpsychiatric physicians to treat pain, but as jail psychiatrists pain is not something we treat. Although nortriptyline causes less drowsiness than amitriptyline, it still can cause drowsiness in people who take it, even if they do not have a mental illness, so it is a drug.

This medication will destabilize someone with true bipolar disorder. It should be avoided in such cases.

It can be fatal in overdose. Nortriptyline should not be used in a jail environment.

Olanzapine (Zyprexa) is a second-generation antipsychotic. It was developed to replicate clozapine's efficacy without replicating clozapine's propensity to cause agranulocytosis. It succeeded partially in the former and fully in the latter. Unfortunately, it replicated clozapine's deleterious side effects: weight gain; obesity; type 2 diabetes, even in the absence of obesity; dyslipidemia; hyperprolactinemia (and you thought that only risperidone caused that). Unfortunately, olanzapine did not emulate clozapine's success in curing otherwise impossible-to-treat psychoses, though it is an excellent antipsychotic.

Olanzapine can be used to treat the psychoses

of schizophrenia and psychotic mania. Olanza-pine should not be used for its side effects, its tranquilizing or sedating effects. Do not use this heavy-duty medication to treat such problems as anxiety and/or insomnia. For one thing, we jailhouse shrinks do not treat those conditions. For another, you could cause a metabolic syn-drome while chasing symptoms. For yet another thing, you could cause the inmate to experience akathisia; and akathisia can lead to suicidal behav-ior. Finally, you may cause tardive dyskinesia— all because an inmate does not adjust well to his or her surroundings. First of all, do no harm.

NB—It may be that combining olanzapine with the opiate antagonist **samidorphan** (not available in the US yet) will mitigate olanzapine-induced weight gain. It does not reduce olanza-pine's antipsychotic effect. This combination is in Phase III trials as this book is being published.

Opiate (no psychiatric indications) I hope by now that you know the mental health providers do not treat pain. Opiates have no psychiatric indications. Opiates should not be used by mental health providers in a jail.

Further, recent research suggests that opiates do not treat chronic pain. Certainly people dependent on opiates experience pain as part of withdrawal and detox—even if there is no under-lying physical cause for pain. This suggests that people with physical conditions are not experienc-ing trouble from their physical ailment(s), but are withdrawing from opiates. An alternative treatment for pain would be the combination of ibuprofen and acetaminophen.

Orphenadrine (generic) is an anticholinergic analog of diphenhydramine. Originally used against Parkinsonism, it is now used mainly to treat muscle spasms. It is mentioned here because it has been abused.

Oxcarbazepine (Trileptal) was brought to market as an anticonvulsant similar to carbamazepine. In fact it is a derivative of carbamazepine. Apparently, it can treat the mood abnormalities seen in mania. When you do use it, you should know that it requires a dose that is 50% greater than that of carbamazepine. That explains the pill sizes: 300mg etc. Do note that use of this medicine is associated with hyponatremia in 17% of cases. Check your BMP's.

Oxcarbazepine has not been tested in treating people with ND-PAE, IED or other conditions marked by anger. It might be helpful for those conditions, reducing a person's anger and propensity to fight. Time will tell.

Paliperidone (Invega) is a second-generation antipsychotic related to risperidone. Unfortunately, it shares with risperidone its propensity to cause hyperprolactinemia, in addition to the expected incidence of diabetes, weight gain, dyslipidemia etc. It is available as a depot injection, but if the injection ends up in fatty tissue, it does not work. This medication is not likely to be on your jail's formulary.

Paroxetine (Paxil) is an SSRI. It is quite useful in treating depression and anxiety. This is one of the medications with a discontinuation syndrome that can produce flu-like symptoms if the medication is suddenly stopped. Although the syndrome can feel severe, it will not kill, as a withdrawal syndrome will. This is a good medicine to use for the depressive symptoms that accompany PTSD, but it does cause weight gain in some patients.

Perphenazine (Trilafon) is a first-generation antipsychotic that works pretty well in reducing or eliminating psychosis. This medication may or may not be on your formulary, depending on the machinations of generic manufacturers. There is a perphenazine-amitriptyline combination (Triavil, Etrafon) but the addition of a TCA makes this medication inappropriate for jail use. Stick with perphenazine and an SSRI.

Pimavanserin (Nuplazid) is an antipsychotic that has been approved to treat delusions and hallucinations in Parkinson's Disease. Do remember that the hallucinations of PD are usually visual, which is unusual in psychiatric disorders.

But time will tell if it maintains its FDA approval.

Pimozide (Orap) is a first-generation antipsychotic. It was brought to the US as an orphan drug for the treatment of Tourette's syndrome. However, it has the acute side effects of akathisia, dystonia and other EPS symptoms, as well as a prolonged QTc interval. Longer term, it can produce tardive dyskinesia. It is probably not on your jail's formulary.

Pramipexole (Mirapex) is used in PD and

RLS. In psychiatry, it is experimental.

Prazosin (Minipress) is a medicine first marketed as an antihypertensive. It is a so-called alpha-1 blocker (adrenergic system). Prazosin has found use as a treatment for PTSD, allegedly reducing the frequency and intensity of traumatic nightmares. However, some studies contradict this usage, so the usefulness of this medication for psychiatry is uncertain. Prazosin is not well tolerated in patients without hypertension. It can produce symptoms of postural hypotension and fainting, so ask about lightheadedness when standing up. Prazosin may not be on your formulary. It may be available only to medical specialists.

Pregabalin (Lyrica) is an anticonvulsant that is used to treat pain. It may be used to treat anxiety with a mechanism similar to benzodiazepines. It can also produce addiction. Psychiatrists do not prescribe pregabalin in jails.

Promethazine (generic) is an antihistamine known for its soporific properties. It is also used for abuse under the names "purple syrup," "syrup" and "lean."

Propranolol (Inderal) was first marketed as an antihypertensive, a "beta blocker" acting by competing with adrenaline at the end organ (beta-adrenergic) receptors. Because propranolol crosses the blood-brain barrier, general medical clinicians tend to prefer other beta-blockers such as metoprolol, which do not cross the blood-brain barrier.

Because propranolol crosses the blood-brain barrier, it has been used as a non-BZD method of treating anxiety. Outside jail, some people take a little propranolol before going onstage. But when used for anxiety, it is still a drug: it will relax anybody.

Propranolol is also useful in the treatment of essential tremor and other physiologic tremors. Since those tremors often do not always include a psychological component, they can often be reduced with a beta-blocker which does not cross the blood-brain barrier, like metoprolol. Here is a clear example of a tremor which does not indicate an inner state of anxiety.

Cases involving tremor should be referred to the general medical specialist. If the tremor is an essential tremor, a medical doctor can treat it. If the tremor indicates the inmate is in withdrawal, the medical specialist should certainly see the inmate and manage the case.

Propranolol can be used as part of the treatment for withdrawal from a number of substances. But best to let the general medical specialist manage the case.

There is one psychiatric indication for propranolol, and that is akathisia. But when you use it, "start low and go slow." Ask the inmate about symptoms of postural hypotension (lightheadedness, fainting) as you monitor and increase the dose. You should probably start at 10mg BID. Remember that if the inmate is diabetic, you cannot use propranolol: since adrenaline is the signaling mechanism for hypoglycemia, anything that blocks the signal—like propranolol—could leave the inmate open to hypoglycemia. In such cases, don't order propranolol.

Quetiapine (Seroquel) is a drug, heroin in a pill. Lots of heroin addicts love it, and make it the first thing they ask for when they come to jail. Most prisons, jails and forensic hospitals have removed it from their formularies, forbidding its use. Diversion is a huge problem with quetiapine. Inmates really like their drugs. Some people use it as a sleeping pill. Like chlorpromazine, it can sedate someone with ADHD.

As a second-generation antipsychotic, quetiapine is a poor antipsychotic. It requires dosing throughout the day and you need to use twice the dose of chlorpromazine to get an antipsychotic effect. Therefore, it is half as potent as chlorpromazine.

This is a drug, because it will calm anyone down. When you are using it for anxiety or sleep, you are exposing the person to dyslipidemia, obesity and type II diabetes, even in the absence of obesity. The diabetes can linger for years. We saw a case where a 19-year-old took quetiapine for three months. Five years later, he was still had diabetes.

Almost as bad, a person can become addicted to it, and have a withdrawal syndrome similar to that of opiates. In at least one case, an inmate has had genuine physical withdrawal symptoms as measured by a blood pressure cuff.

That said, quetiapine can be used on the

outside to help treat the depressive symptoms of a mixed manic-depressive episode of genuine bipolar disorder. The use of quetiapine for "bipolar disorder" (dysthymia etc.) is a mistake. With so problematic a drug, using it seems almost cruel. Quetiapine should not be prescribed in a jail environment.

Ramelteon (Rozerem) is a melatonin analog. Because it is used for sleep, it is not used in jails. Some studies show some efficacy in delirium, however, so ramelteon or something like it may eventually be used to treat demented patients with delirium instead of antipsychotics, which in many cases will kill them.

Retigabine European name for ezogabine.

Riluzole has been approved to treat ALS. Its use in psychiatric disorders is experimental.

Rimonabant is an inverse agonist for the cannabinoid receptor CB1. At the time of this writing, it is approved nowhere, so don't prescribe it.

Risperidone (Risperdal) is the first of the second-generation antipsychotics. It has enough similarity with first-generation antipsychotics that it could be thought of as a 1.5-generation antipsychotic. Risperidone can be given alone, with fewer first-generation side effects than you would expect. With or without side effect meds, risperidone is an effective antipsychotic. It can be given in doses as low as 0.25mg to 1mg with good effect, though a dose of 2-3mg is used more often. You will frequently see this medication prescribed BID, but it can be given once a day.

Surprisingly, the upper limit on dosing is 16mg per day (!). But you would not need to treat with such doses in a jail setting.

Probably the most prominent side effect of risperidone is hyperprolactinemia, or "man boobs." But risperidone is hardly the only second-generation antipsychotic to produce this side effect. In addition to producing more EPS side effects than other second-generation antipsychotics, risperidone can cause the usual panoply of diabetes, obesity, dyslipidemia etc. Despite all of that, risperidone is the go-to antipsychotic when you treat inmates.

Risperidone is also available as biweekly and monthly injectable forms.

St. John's Wort (Hypericum perforatum) is an herbal preparation used to treat depression, similar to SSRI's. Because it is not standardized by the FDA, it is not provided in hospitals, jails etc. If someone has recently used SJW, you should wait 2 weeks or so to start an SSRI or SNRI to prevent the possibility of a serotonin syndrome.

SAMe (S-Adenosyl methionine) is marketed as a nutritional supplement to treat depression. Because it is not standardized by the FDA, it is not provided in hospitals, jails, etc. If someone has recently used SAMe, you should wait 2 weeks or so to start an SSRI or SNRI to prevent the possibility of a serotonin syndrome.

Samidorphan See olanzapine.

Sertraline (Zoloft) was the second SSRI. It has been used successfully in the treatment of depression, anxiety, PMD and PMS. Dosage rages from 25mg QAM to 200mg QAM, with 50mg treating most people. Sertraline was found to help the depression associated with PTSD in an early study, so it has frequently been used for that condition. Sertraline seems to cause nausea, diarrhea and other GI side effects marginally more often than other SSRI's. Also, I have seen a mild SSRI discontinuation syndrome with this medication at 100mg QD. Sertraline has the interesting property of causing drowsiness in about 20% of people who take it. This drowsiness comes about 5 hours after taking the medication. Sertraline causes wakefulness in about as many people who take it. Thus, you would start it QAM but it can be prescribed at HS if an inmate says the medicine is making her drowsy.

Sertraline was extensively marketed to FP's when it first came out. Thus, the company avoided directly competing with fluoxetine. The main import of this is that for years after, FP's used sertraline as their go-to SSRI. Overall, it is a good medication, and it should be a routine part of your armamentarium in the jail setting.

SNRI (Selective Norepinephrine-Serotonin Reuptake Inhibitors; desvenlafaxine, duloxetine, mirtazapine and venlafaxine) A term formed analogously to SSRI's, which came first. This is a class of medications which have in common an ability to inhibit the reabsorption of serotonin and norepinephrine in CNS synapses. These medications have side effects similar to the SSRI's.

These medications will destabilize someone with true bipolar disorder; SNRI's should be avoided in such cases. Also, all SNRI's increase BP, so keep that in mind.

SSRI (Selective Serotonin Reuptake Inhibitors; citalopram, escitalopram, fluoxetine, fluvoxamine, paroxetine and sertraline) is a class of medications which have in common an ability to inhibit the reabsorption of serotonin in CNS synapses. They are used to treat depression, anxiety, anger and depressive symptoms. They are used to treat the same symptoms when they come from PTSD. Prominent side effects include GI disturbance, sexual and urinary dysfunction and an odd daze-like sedation. Luckily, most of these effects are mild, and none of these affect the majority of people who take SSRI's.

The nausea that afflicts some people is usually transient, and can be avoided by ramping up the medication to the desired therapeutic dose rather than suddenly starting at that dose. If a person cannot tolerate an SSRI, usually another can be found which the inmate can tolerate.

These medications are often successful in "bipolar" disorder. These can be used—albeit carefully—in true bipolar disorder, if a mood stabilizer or an antipsychotic is prescribed concurrently with the antidepressant.

When an inmate claims that she has tried them all, including SNRI's, bupropion and buspirone and none work, do not be afraid to tell her that this situation is unfortunate: you have nothing further to try, and she needs psycho-therapy. Under no circumstances break down and give her a drug. If you do, then all the inmates will be coming to your office and turning on the waterworks again and again until they get the drugs they crave.

Sufentanil (Dsuvia) is a synthetic opioid 10 times more powerful than its analog fentanyl and 1000 times more potent than morphine. Similar to carfentanyl, it has no place in a psychiatric practice (on the same day the FDA approved this for pain, they disapproved an opioid "treatment" for depression).

Temazepam (Restoril) is a benzodiazepine, marketed as a sleeping pill. It carries all the baggage of a benzodiazepine, and like all benzodi-azepines, disrupts one's sleep architecture. For this reason, it probably should be prescribed only on a spot basis in your outside practice. It has no place in jails.

Testosterone has been used as an antide-pressant, but using the male hormone this way is experimental. However, some day . . .

Thioridazine (Mellaril) is a low-potency first-generation antipsychotic about as strong and about as sedating as chlorpromazine. It has a black box warning in re- prolonged QTc intervals on the EKG. Thioridazine is not prescribed much these days. It is probably not on your jail's formulary.

Thiothixene (Navane) A first-generation antipsychotic with antidepressant properties. This was used for schizoaffective disorder and psychotic depression as well as for more common psychoses.

Tianeptine is a TCA that is also a μ-opioid agonist. It is not legally available in the US, but abuse happens. Deaths from overdose have occurred. Michigan recently classified tianeptine as a Schedule II controlled substance after a series of overdoses. Because this is a TCA, it has no place in jails.

Tizanidine (Zanaflex) The VA said that it had "discovered that . . . can be used for treatment of symptoms associated with PTSD." This medication is apparently better tolerated than prazosin, which is an alpha-1 antagonist. You can see that any treatment for PTSD would be very important for the VA. At the time of this writing, the VA was unsuccessful in its search for further development. Too bad, but it will sedate anyone who takes it, so it is a drug. Drugs have no place in jails. See also MDMA.

Topiramate (Topamax) Despite what psychiatrists would like, topiramate is NOT a mood-stabilizer. Every time it has been tested in an RCT on true bipolar patients it failed to separate from placebo. It is an anticonvulsant. It acts as a prophylactic against migraines. It will cause weight loss, sometimes a dramatic weight loss (100 lbs. in a year). Topiramate will also make a person without psychiatric illness feel relaxed, so it is a drug. Topiramate has no official psychiatric indication, so it has no place in a psychiatric practice in jails.

Tramadol (Ultram) is used to treat pain. It has most of its action as a mu-opioid agonist, lesser effects on kappa and o-opioid receptors. This drug may have antidepressant effects—it can induce mania—but those effects are over-shadowed by its opioid effects. Officially, no psychiatric indications.

Trazodone (Desyrel) is an antidepressant—and a good one—in the antidepressant dose range of 300-600mg/day. These days, trazodone is more known as a sleeping pill in doses of 10-50mg HS. This medication will sedate most people—even those without psychiatric illness—so it is a drug. Also, it can lengthen the QTc interval, and that requires monitoring. If you stop a large dose of trazodone suddenly, you can get a discontinuation syndrome. Trazodone is not prescribed in jails.

Triazolam (Halcion) is a BZD known for prominent amnesic effects. As a BZD, it is not prescribed in jails.

Trifluoperazine (Stelazine) is a first-generation antipsychotic, the first high potency antipsychotic. It is about 25 times as potent as chlorpromazine.

Trihexyphenidyl (Artane) is an antiparkinsonian medication. It has anticholinergic effects. It should be given BID, because of its relatively short duration of action. It may or may not be on your jail's formulary.

Tricyclic Antidepressant (TCA; amitriptyline, clomipramine, cyclobenzaprine [not an antidepressant], desipramine, doxepin, imipramine,

nortriptyline, protriptyline, tianeptine and trimipramine). TCA's were the second generation of
antidepressants. They are still used for major
depression: in their prime it was said they were
about 80% effective for that condition. One
problem was that, even when these medications
were used under supervision, various issues
would come up—postural hypotension, cardio-
toxicity, unexpected drowsiness, weight gain,
fatal overdoses—so GP's would avoid using
them; hence the utility of SSRI's, which require a
lot less supervision. Even when these medications were used properly, they were a leading
cause of death from overdose. They were not to
be trifled with. TCA's should not be used in jails.

Trimipramine (Surmontil) is a TCA that was
used because of its purported soporific and
anxiolytic properties. In its heyday it was not as
popular as other TCA's. As a TCA it should not be
prescribed in a jail setting.

Typical Antipsychotics This is an unfortunate name for the first-generation of antipsychotic
medications. The name refers to the fact that
these medicines produce EPS side effects. "Typical" antipsychotics target DA receptors to combat
psychosis. Studies have found that just as many
schizophrenic patients like the first-generation
antipsychotic medications as like the second-
generation medications. These chemicals are considered neurotoxic now. First-generation antipsychotics should be used only when second-
generation medications cause adverse effects, or

when the inmate does better on the old meds. They are also called 'neuroleptics.'

Valproic Acid (Depakene) is an anticonvulsant that is closely related to divalproex (see).

Valbenazine (Ingrezza) has been approved to treat tardive dyskinesia.

Vitamin C (ascorbic acid) is a treatment for scurvy. This should interest psychiatrists because the first symptom of scurvy is depression. Although inmates are normally provided with balanced diets that include all essential vitamins, an inmate's dietary preferences may lead him into a deficiency of Vitamin C. Just keep this one tucked in the back of your mind.

Venlafaxine (Effexor) is an antidepressant that also reduces complaints of anxiety. At lower doses it is an SSRI. At higher doses venlafaxine affects both the serotonin and norepinephrine receptors, so it becomes an SNRI. It is not sedating, so it is not a drug. Venlafaxine can treat neuropathic pain and seems to have a positive effect in some cases of ADHD. When venlafaxine was first available in its IR (immediate release) form it had to be given in divided doses, at least TID. Its nickname among competing drug reps was "ineffexor." When the XR form was released, that stopped. Venlafaxine became a once-a-day medication and was quite effective in depression. Venlafaxine has indications for depression, generalized anxiety disorder (GAD), social anxiety disorder (social phobia), and panic disorder, with or without agoraphobia. Some studies show it stops hot flashes, too. It is actually less expensive these days to treat with venlafaxine XR once a day, especially when you consider the nurse's time.

Three caveats: If you suddenly stop venlafaxine, you will frequently see people complaining of a discontinuation syndrome. This can be quite unpleasant, though harmless, with flu-like symptoms, headache and an "electric shock in the brain" sensation. Also, venlafaxine can destabilize a case of true bipolar disorder; so, when you have or suspect that, you will have to avoid using venlafaxine. Finally, as with all SNRI's, venlafaxine can elevate blood pressure.

Vilazodone (Viibryd) is an antidepressant, one which affects a number of neurotransmitters. Vilazodone's claim to fame may be its sparing of sexual functioning. It is too new to be on the formulary at most jails.

Vortioxetine (Trintellix, Brintellix) is an antidepressant. It acts as a serotonin modulator. It is new, so it is probably not on your formulary.

Ziprasidone (Geodon) is a second generation antipsychotic. Despite that, akathisia is not an unusual side effect. A more common side effect is the lengthening of the QTc interval. When ziprasidone was first proposed, the manufacturers of competing medications pointed this out to the FDA, which studied the phenomenon. It turned out that thioridazine produced QTc twice as often. We had used that medication for decades without knowing about this. Although thioridazine got the black box warning and ziprasidone did not, it is wise to get an EKG when you start treatment, another partway through dose escalation, and another soon after reaching the highest dose you will be prescribing. Luckily, EKG's are fairly easy to get in jails, with the printout normally including the QTc interval in its readout. The QTc should not exceed 450ms. This medication may or may not be on your jail's formulary.

Zaleplon (Sonata) is a sleeping pill. As such, it is not appropriate for jails.

Zolpidem (Ambien) is a sleeping pill. As such it is not appropriate for jails.

Zopiclone is not sold in the US. It is a sleeping pill, and thus not appropriate for jails.

Appendix MI
Military History

Getting a correct military history is not as important as it used to be. In the past, people faked wild military histories and PTSD to get drugs. Now, as even the VA recognizes that there are no drug cures for actual PTSD, it seems to be less of an issue in jails these days. However, if MDMA is approved for PTSD, this may change.

Getting a history can help with treatment using medications or psychotherapy. In particular you should ask a high school graduate if he or she tried to join a military service. If the person failed to get in, was it because he or she already had felonies? Or did the person take the exam and fail, thus showing you that the person probably lacked the intellectual capacity for armed services? This probably places your inmate in the BIF range or lower.

But maybe your HS grad says he or she was in the military. If true, it indicates that your inmate had a degree of psychosocial functioning that is unusual among inmates.

Army

After one has been recruited into the Army one is shipped to a Basic Training post, there to undergo Basic Combat Training (BCT), often referred to as "Basic." Note that Army personnel are assigned to "posts," which may be at Forts or Camps. Other services call their facilities "bases."

Today's BCT posts at Ft Jackson, SC, Ft Leonard Wood, MO, or Ft Sill, OK, are the posts that have gender-integrated BCT. Posts that provide male-only BCT are Ft Benning GA and Ft Knox KY.

A recruit may be discharged from the Army during BCT due to misconduct, unsatisfactory performance or medical conditions. The medical conditions can be pre-existing conditions, or problems that revealed themselves only during training. When I served at a basic training post, people would periodically crack up under the stress of training. We had learned of a so-called 'immigrant syndrome' in our psychiatric training; of people coming to the new world and overwhelmed with stress, abruptly becoming psychotic. This appeared to be the same phenomenon. Certainly, we saw manic episodes provoked by BCT.

After BCT comes Advanced Individual Training (AIT). There are various schools in the Army, where recruits learn their military trades. Here is where they earn their MOS.

After AIT comes Active Duty. A soldier can be stationed at any of the above sites. There are other duty stations, however. They may be put into a position they have not trained for. Regardless, the position dictates the MOS.

An enlistment normally lasts 3 years. Some people engage in 6-year enlistments. Enlisted ranks run from Private (E-1 and E-2), Private First Class (PFC, E-3), Corporal (E-4), Sergeant (E-5), to higher ranks of sergeant (E-6 to E-9). An interviewer would expect a man to reach E-5 by the end of a 6-year tour in the Army. Asking about the discharge rank will give you information: if a discharge rank is too low, it suggests that the serviceman was "busted," or reduced in rank during his service.

If a soldier is disabled and discharged for his disability, he is placed on the Temporary Disability Retired List (TDRL) for up to five years. When the Army puts people on TDRL status for psychiatric reasons, it seems that it expects them to be permanently disabled. At about 5 years they are reevaluated. When an inmate describes this process, he has usually had a legitimate disability discharge from the Army.

Some inmates will flat out tell you they had a dishonorable discharge or left on OTH (other than honorable) status. Some of these inmates still receive services from the VA.

Marines (USMC)

The Marines begin their training with "boot camp" at Parris Island NC or San Diego CA. After this, they will enter a School of Infantry (SOI) at Camp Lejeune, NC, or Camp Pendleton, CA. Following this they scatter to various sites for training in their specialties.

Navy

Enlisted personnel in the Navy are known as sailors. The U.S. Navy used to train people in Florida, in San Diego, CA, and at the Great Lakes facility. Since 1999, the Navy has done their boot camp only at the Great Lakes, Illinois (GLI) facility. Following boot camp sailors scatter to various Advanced Schools ("A-schools"). The SEAL school is in San Diego, for example. NB—if an inmate tells you he was a Marine SEAL, he is lying: SEAL's are sailors only.

Air Force (USAF)

Enlisted personnel in the Air Force are known as airmen, even if they are women. USAF Basic Military Training (BMT) occurs at the Lackland Air Force Base (AFB) in San Antonio, Texas. After BMT, airmen scatter to various schools for specialty training, which may take up to 2 years.

Fake History

Back when inmates were of an age that they could claim to be Viet Nam vets, they did so. They would come in with wild tales of incursions in North Viet Nam, of going out and getting cocaine leaves, etc. Funny thing though: their exploits were always "I can't tell you about it." So why talk at all?

They described SEAL training at a Marine base (SEAL's are in the Navy). They never seemed to remember their MOS. Legitimate members of the Armed services almost always remembers the title and the number of their MOS (Military Occupational Specialty) even decades after they served. Also, they tend to remember the units they served with.

People who have served in an armed service will give you a history where detail is combined with some skipping over the boring parts—just like real life. And with a true history, you can dig down for details and get them. But when a guy tells you that he was in the Army and served at our embassy in Iran in the 1980's and in Afghanistan in the 1990's, well ... we didn't have an embassy in Iran in the 1980's or Afghanistan in the 1990's; and it is the Marine Corps who provide embassy guards, not the Army.

But as usual, fakers are trying to score drugs. They go away disappointed if all you can give them is sertraline and buspirone.

Appendix PA
Panic Attacks

Panic attacks can occur spontaneously. Panic attacks can be a reaction to a phobic situation: driving over a bridge or meeting a group of people. Panic attacks may wake an inmate from sleep. Panic attacks are frightening, mimicking MI's. They are dramatic, and can provoke a medical staff into heroics. Right. In health class, you learn to put a condom on a banana but you learn nothing of normal physiology.

A panic attack is a person's reaction to adrenaline. Adrenaline is our alarm hormone. It is the body's way of getting you ready to handle danger. In order to get your muscles ready to respond, you first feel a need to breathe. So, shortness of breath is adrenaline's way of leading you to gulp in air. Then you must push blood that is full of oxygen to the muscles, so your heart pounds. The blood moving through your arteries and your muscles processing that oxygen make heat. You feel hot all over, so hairs rise up and you sweat, shedding the excess heat. You are aroused, which is the whole point. You are ready for danger.

The shortness of breath you feel in a panic attack is a lie. Look at your hands. The palms are pink or are pink under the pigment. Your nail-beds are pink. Your tongue and the inside of your mouth are pink. You can only get that color if your tissues are full of oxygen. If a person has a panic attack and she is taken to the medical department. The person with a panic attack usually has a blood oxygen approaching 100%. You can demonstrate this with a pulse oximeter.

If your muscles cramp, it is because you are hyperventilating, blowing your CO_2 away.

A panic attack is a person's reaction to adrenaline. If you were driving and just missed hitting a concrete abutment by a couple of inches, you would have shortness of breath, your heart would be pounding, you would be sweating and you would feel hot. You would be exhibiting all the symptoms of a panic attack, but none of the symptoms would surprise you: it's just a normal response to danger, after all.

What scares the person into having a panic attack is the she does not know where the adrenaline is coming from. Worse: she might not know that her symptoms are a normal response to adrenaline. It is your job to explain where the symptoms come from. The inmate is in jail. She is surrounded by dangerous predators—other inmates. Her life outside is going on without her. She is having scary dreams and wakes up afraid, and then the panic attacks proceed.

With proper counseling, an inmate can learn to weather the alarm storm. If she does not get enabled by well-meaning healthcare profession-als eager to "treat" this condition she will notice that the panic attack burns itself out in a few minutes. After a while, she can learn to master herself and the incidence of panic attacks will fade into nothingness.

But if the panic attacks satisfy her need to be the center of attention or provide other secondary gain, then the incidence of these attacks will resist treatment. The person should be in therapy. But beyond providing an SSRI, you should not chase the panic symptoms trying to snuff them out. They won't snuff.

Appendix PT
PTSD

(See also the PTSD section of Chapter 5.)

PTSD is classically represented by a triad of symptom clusters: re-experiencing the traumatic events, avoiding traumatic reminders, and a persistent sense of threat, including hyper-vigilance and excessive startle response.

Lawyers have a general metaphor: the thin-skulled plaintiff. What they mean is that a knock on the head that is nothing to a normal person, may crack the skull of the unusually sensitive person. That person still gets to sue.

Just so, injuries that would be nothing to some people become hideous traumas to others.

War departments have known about PTSD — variously named—since the US Civil War in the 1860's. The French developed a form of psycho-therapy for some sufferers during World War I. The American War Department used hypnosis during and after World War II. But nothing was completely satisfactory for war trauma.

Around the 1990's, researchers discovered that people with certain kinds of pre-existing problems who entered the armed services were more prone to develop PTSD than their comrades who had comparable wartime experiences. Those preexisting problems? A history of molest-ation, rape and substance abuse, for example.

Each problem standing alone is enough to make someone more prone to develop PTSD. Sound like our population?

The diagnostic criteria for PTSD have changed through the years, but the basic symptoms include intrusive thoughts, and reenactments of the trauma in nightmares and emotional responses. The intrusive thoughts seem to lie in ambush, waiting to jump out and surprise (ambush) the victim at any turn.

Traumatic nightmares are a special kind of nightmare. We are used to nightmares that focus on a theme, like running away from dangerous people, etc. Traumatic nightmares, on the other hand, focus on specific events that traumatized the person. Inmates will usually tell you what their nightmares are about.

The emotional responses vary. Some people with PTSD experience emotional numbing. They may have numbing of their memories of the event. They may feel numbness in their interactions with others. For example, children who have been traumatized by urban violence may grow up to join gangs and commit . . . urban violence.

Other people may experience hyperarousal. They may have come to fear groups of people and exhibit phobic responses, complaining of nervousness that their fellow inmates represent a threat to them.

The VA has struggled over 50 years to discover medications to treat PTSD. They found no chemical treatments for PTSD. SSRI's and SNRI's may be helpful for the depression that accompanies most cases of PTSD. Antipsychotics may be useful if PTSD provokes a psychosis. But it is important to note that antipsychotics do NOT reduce the nightmares of PTSD.

Types of Traumas

Traumas to teens and adults may be single or multiple. The traumas suffered by soldiers at war tend to be part of a string of traumas. On the other hand, a rape, or a robbery or the explosion of an IED is a single-episode trauma.

Traumas might be physical or psychological. A physical trauma might be a rape or a stabbing or a gunshot wound. Generally, if there is a threat to the victim's life, it is more likely that she will experience a PTSD. If an IED explodes, there is often a head trauma. Where there is a head trauma, the victim is more likely to experience PTSD.

A psychological trauma might involve a soldier coming into a warehouse in Bosnia and finding hundreds of bodies hung like meat. It might involve finding your father or mother dead of an accidental heroin overdose. The sudden horror seems to stay with people. Seeing a motor vehicle accident where there are fatalities does not have the same intimacy of horror as experiencing the MVA yourself, perhaps losing a brother or a fiancé in the process. Again, these are single-episode traumas.

One surprising aspect of the trauma that can cause PTSD: perps can develop PTSD, especially perps who were traumatized in childhood. People who kill others, people who cause others to suffer, can develop PTSD as much as their victims.

Traumas that occur in childhood

Children are small and vulnerable. Adults who have been set up to watch over them, may beat them or molest them, sometimes over protracted periods. It is interesting the way these traumas play out. Sometimes kids experience the most horrific trauma and develop not a PTSD picture, but dysthymia and borderline personality disorder. This is why some therapists consider BPD to be "Complex PTSD."

ICD-11 finally will have a code for Complex PTSD. It will feature the normal Big Three of PTSD in addition to disturbances in self-organization (DSO)—disturbances in relationships, negative self-concept, affective dysregulation.

When children grow up to have PTSD, the symptoms appear to be just like those of adult-onset PTSD, though there may be some ascertainment bias here. As previously noted, some consider BPD to be a form of PTSD, albeit a complex one.

Single-episode traumas suffered in childhood may involve having your parent killed in front of you. They may involve a rape or a kidnapping. Sometimes children—especially boys—might react violently. Unfortunately, our predecessors often treated this reaction formation with antipsychotics rather than counseling. When told "Don't just stand there, do something," they did, drugging the kid up rather than letting him express his grief in catharsis.

The problem with traumas experienced in childhood, is that it breaks the bubble of false invulnerability that we all wear about ourselves. It creates a "Sitting Duck Syndrome" (part of the title of an important paper by Richard Klufft, MD). The person is seen thereafter to be eternally vulnerable. Perps pick up on this and prey upon them, visiting more trauma on those who were traumatized when young. If you have ever wondered why certain people seem to pick up way more than their share of traumas across their lives, this is why.

Responses

People respond in varying ways to trauma. When the trauma does not involve an assault on the victim and does not involve injury to the victim, it is less likely to cause PTSD. PTSD is not an inevitable consequence of traumas. Sometimes people simply have a bad day.

Associated Disorders

A recent study found that more than half of people with combat-related PTSD also had sleep apnea. Because people with sleep apnea generally have treatment-resistant psychiatric conditions, it would seem straightforward to treat the sleep apnea and then wait to see if further treatment is necessary. It is not yet clear if people with non-combat trauma also have sleep apnea, but it seems like a good avenue of inquiry to follow if the inmate has PTSD.

Substance use disorders also occur commonly in cases of PTSD, whether combat-related or from civilian trauma, and whether the trauma is from a single event, a few events, or recurrent events. A person using substances will not be ready for treatment until after the detox phase is finished: he is still too wrapped up in his drugs to attend to anything else.

Nightmares

Why do we have nightmares in PTSD?

Nightmares are a species of dream, dreams that wake you up before you can finish them. Dreams seem to be a way of extracting guidance or "rules of thumb" from the details of our lives. In dreams we juxtapose various elements seeing how they do or do not fit together. Nightmares are like this, but so intense that they wake us. Note that PTSD-related nightmares are not "night terrors." Night terrors are a non-REM problem, usually seen in children. Nightmares occur during REM sleep. Theme-related nightmares are not a concern here: dreams of pursuit by faceless bad people are regular dreams. Dreams that re-create the specific events when and where the inmate suffered trauma—those are PTSD-related nightmares.

Dreams could be considered as one of a mind's problem-solving mechanisms. But why do we have nightmares in PTSD? Nightmares may continue, repeating until you learn the lessons.

Treatment Considerations

PTSD is a psychological injury requiring psychological treatment. In a jail, the mental health department will not be able to provide the kind of psychotherapy needed to fully help someone with PTSD. So how do you treat it? SSRI's will only treat the depression associated with PTSD. A clue for treatment may be found in EMDR. EMDR is a successful treatment for PTSD. It has found success when there is overt trauma and success when the trauma is covert hidden by layers of neurosis.

Another treatment may be the club drug MDMA, known a "ecstasy." It is in Phase III trials for use in treatment-resistant PTSD. If this is approved, expect inmates to clamor for it.

There are two considerations here: inmates who are not documented as getting MDMA from a psychiatrist on entry to jail, can be dismissed as lying or not ready (there is likely to be a previous treatment requirement). Second, as a drug of abuse, MDMA may not be allowed at your jail.

When people get pensions for having PTSD, you cannot expect any chemical to work.

So what does work?

From its beginning in the late 1980's, EMDR has been the classic treatment for PTSD. However, since that time it has spread out to find the hidden traumas of childhood that can lead to distress in adulthood. The basis of EMDR is to find memories that have not been processed properly and reprocess them. The success of EMDR therapists in finding those hidden traumas goes a long way to explaining why it works so well. For example, a woman I know in a mountain state was unable to drive down hills due to a fear of heights. In her area this was particularly disabling. EMDR sessions allowed this woman to abandon her acrophobia. Now she is able to drive in mountainous terrain.

One technique used in EMDR involves separating the sufferer from the traumatic memory. This allows a person to see herself being traumatized (the separation attenuates the pain). This technique suggests a method for coping with nightmares. Imagine a sports team looking at a game film. There they are, sitting at a table in the present looking at themselves in the past. They use it to critique their playing. We can use it for more than that.

Dreams can be guided. If you consciously decide on how dreams will work out, research shows your dreams will follow your waking decisions. So you can instruct the traumatized person to recognize when she is entering her past during her dream and to divert that dream to an imaginary screen. In the meantime, she is diverting herself to a seat from which to watch the dream on the screen. She can look and have feelings. She can feel disgusted, sad and angry, but not afraid. She will not feel afraid, because she is alive. She has survived the trauma. The person on the screen—her past self—did not know what was coming, so she felt afraid. The person watching the traumatic experience unfold is free to observe side details like how the perp got her into a space where he could traumatize her in the first place. She is free to follow the details because she is not afraid she will die. She can learn the lesson, whatever it is.

This is not always a helpful tool. But some inmates can profit greatly from it. One veteran in particular found it very helpful. He remembered a bunch of soldiers who went into Mogadishu, where they were badly shot up. Using the technique, he was able to look at them, thinking "that man survived, that man died and that man we medevacked out"—plus one guy (his past self) was scared spitless about all of them. The man having the nightmare was finally able to stop his PTSD.

The important thing to note here is that this technique involves coaching an inmate to do the therapy on himself. You will not have time to do PTSD therapy with all who need it. Nor will you have time to coach everyone who could use some coaching on coping with nightmares. This technique might be helpful for a selected few, however.

PTSD can result in depression, anxiety and social avoidance (social phobia). A rational treatment of the former might be an SSRI like sertraline. A rational treatment of the anxiety might be buspirone. If the inmate is frightened of others (social phobia) you might choose venlafaxine as an antidepressant.

Prazosin is controversial: it was introduced first as an antihypertensive and does cause hypotension. Worse, it promotes sleep, even in those not mentally ill. This is the kind of medicine best used outside of jails.

Although MDMA is now is Phase III trials for treating PTSD, it may not ever be allowed in jails because of abuse considerations.

We may hear about hydrocortisone in the future because some RCT's support its use in PTSD. But at present, this is still experimental and not to be used in a jail setting.

First of all, do no harm.

Appendix R
Reactive vs
Instrumental

Reactive behavior—acting in response to a stressor, often without thinking first.

Instrumental behavior—doing something to get something.

Reactive behavior. We classically think of mental patients as having 'reactions' to various things. DSM-II, for example, was full of 'reactions.' But today, we think less that a person's response is a reaction to an event, than the symptoms of reaction are part of a pathological system. Yet patients and non-patient people do react to events, good and bad. The concept of reaction formation still has value today. Reaction formation may involve a person's response to acute or repeated trauma. Reactions may involve violence. Reactions may involve secondary gain. An example of that, would be reactions that involve self-injury, frequently self-cutting. Without recognizing it, these people are seeking to release endorphins to calm themselves down. Other responses involve rebelling against the injustices or abuses of the past, transferred to someone in the present, or acting out an old script where the inmate played a part, and the part of the other is transferred to someone in the present. In general, reactions are just that—a person's reacting to something.

Instrumental behaviors are purposeful actions. They may involve self-injury. Those actions are calculated to invoke reactions in caregivers. Often the actions have the intent, like terrorism, of provoking horror. But think about it: IV addicts stick themselves with needles multiple times a day. They often share needles. Do you think that mere self-injury is any kind of an impediment to their behavior?

Instrumental actions are often the actions of predators. There are lots of predators in jails. Many are seeking drugs. But these drug-seeking individuals do not have a mental illness, no matter how much they complain. They really should not be considered patients, since if they were not in jail, they would see no need for a psychiatrist. This is one of the many reasons we call the people we treat "inmates" rather than "patients."

As an example of instrumental behavior, a heroin addict was making time with an attractive female on the ward, but his play for her was interrupted when he finished his withdrawal, and his attending discharged him. So he walked into the parking lot and out to his truck, where he retrieved a hook knife. There he cut himself—two long lacerations on the volar surfaces of each arm, from pit to wrist. Then he walked back into the ER, streaming blood. Of course he was readmitted. Mission accomplished.

Countless times, inmates bang their heads on the wall. Sometimes they are trying to go to sleep or to produce endorphins to calm down; but they also bang their heads to get what they want—to see the Warden for special treatment, or to get to the ER for an evaluation, out of the jail, and where he might score an opiate or call the outside. It is up to the shrink—maybe a psychologist, maybe you—to figure out the difference.

One local jail has difficulty with a particular inmate who likes to cut his arteries, so he can spray his blood and catch the unwary caregiver. In the past, he would sling body fluids; but because he can be prosecuted for aggravated assault when he does that, he switched to cutting himself and squirting blood. For one thing, this horrifies caregivers, especially when he bleeds out copious amounts of blood and comes near death; this is a psychological assault, for one thing. It becomes a physical assault when he attacks someone with his blood. He has not been prosecuted so far for this, because the self-cutting and blood are intrinsically horrifying. More recently, he faked an unending seizure. The nurses correctly diagnosed a pseudoseizure, but the doctor chickened out and prescribed hydroxyzine. This seemed to calm the inmate for a time, and he stopped "seizing" as he waited for the drug to kick in. When it did not, he realized it was not a benzodiazepine, so he resumed his pretense of having a seizure. It continued until he fell asleep. He is infamous in the facility among CO's and healthcare workers. Perhaps because he is a criminal, he seems to enjoy psychologically assaulting others, in addition to using his body to achieve his goal. Call him the poster child for instrumental behavior. Just to be clear: when that inmate is not in jail, he exhibits none of this behavior.

Inmates and patients in situations where they cannot get opiates have been known to injure themselves so they could be sent to a non-corrections hospital. There the staff would treat them with opiates.

Finally, there is instrumental nonbehavior. Occasionally you will come upon a person who claims that he cannot walk. After being assessed at a local ER and found to be malingering, a good medical department will remove all devices like wheelchairs, forcing the person to walk. But what if the inmate can persuade CO's to provide him with a wheelchair? An inmate developed strictures by confining himself to a wheelchair—he was such a good faker that he ended up developing the very condition he pretended. Of course, this is not an intelligent way to get a sentence reduced, but who said inmates were bright? As one CO remarked, "You don't go to jail for doing something smart."

Appendix S Suicidality

One onerous task you will probably not be able to escape is to "clear" a person from suicide precautions.

Suicide precautions in your jail may involve a variety of conditions:

Level 0: Restraint Chair. Psychiatrists usually do not order that this be used. It is a Custody intervention that they may use when an inmate is engaging in instrumental behavior, like cutting himself or hanging himself in full view of an observer.

Level 1: Constant Observation, or 1:1 Observation. Jails will vary in the circumstances they hold such a one. Psychiatrists may order this.

Level 2: Constant Watch, or Q15-minute checks, while the inmate is housed by himself in suicide-resistant circumstances (wearing a suicide-resistant gown known as a "turtle suit" or "chicken suit," no access to blankets, etc.). Psychiatrists may order this.

Level 3: Constant Watch, or Q15-minute checks while the inmate is housed in the company of others (he may have a cellmate or have access to a group) and property. Psychiatrists may order this.

Or a jail may specify a "Suicide Watch," where an inmate is held without clothing in a bare cell. There are many variations.

An observer may be a CO, someone hired for the task, or an inmate worker, depending on the jail.

People are put on 1:1 suicide watch, or "suicide precautions," ostensibly to prevent suicide. But actually, the jail administration wants to stop inmates from suicidal behavior—whether it is a suicide attempt or a suicide gesture. After all, someone pretending to kill himself may succeed by accident. So your task is to figure out how likely it is that someone may "attempt" a "suicidal" act.

The bottom line is that you must assess the likelihood that an inmate will do something to harm himself. Note that you do not care if someone is truly suicidal, but that he will do something to himself.

Companies and researchers have spent a lot of time and effort determining who is actually suicidal, but that is not really your main concern. Your main concern is whether the inmate will act out, and run the risk of killing himself.

When assessing whether someone is suicidal, you must document reasons that hold him on earth, such as a significant other or a child. Shameful charges? If she feels worthless, record that, too. And his impulsivity. If someone feels like living, she is less likely to try to kill herself. If someone is impulsive and has suicidal impulses, he might try to do himself in. An inmate may engage in a suicide gesture to prove to his family or to himself how ashamed he is. As long as the person is in danger, keep him on suicide watch.

One psychologist has found that inmates who commit suicide tend to be angry, dependent or avoidant, and were rejected by someone.

On the contrary, you may see people that have no reason to kill themselves. Yet they are trying to convince you or others that they are willing to kill themselves. They tie something around their necks or cut themselves or take an overdose. They are using their "suicidal" intentions to accomplish something, to pull something off. They are no more suicidal than the man in the moon, yet they will try something as soon as you take them off suicide watch. They might kill themselves by accident. You should keep those people on suicide watch, and in your note explain your reasons for doing so.

The jail may have an alternative for such people, but your first clinical impulse should be to prevent suicidal and "suicidal" acting out.

It is not safe to house a potentially suicidal inmate alone on 15-minute checks if he has access to clothing or anything else he could kill himself with. Either clothe the person in a suicide-resistant gown ("turtle suit" or "chicken suit") or house the inmate with a cellmate on Q15-minute checks. Remember that your jail may not have a suicide-resistant blanket. An inmate can kill himself with a normal blanket.

One can find all sorts of real-world examples. There was a man who was not suicidal, but wanted changes in his circumstances. So he "hung up," thinking the CO would find him while doing his Q15-minute checks. But the officer was detained slightly, and the inmate died. It was an example of poor judgment leading accidentally to a fatal outcome. It is that poor judgment that jails—and you—must protect inmates against.

Another inmate killed himself following a telephone conversation with his parents. Did something they said cause him to hang himself? Or did he have akathisia from haloperidol? The latter case is why psychiatrists should not try to treat detox with antipsychotics.

So, what are your markers?

If he has children, a nonsuicidal inmate will often say (usually loudly) "I wanna live. I got kids!" Recently, a person facing sex charges told me he was thinking of killing himself, and he had three children. I left him on Suicide Watch. Later, after he had thought about it, he was no longer suicidal, and could come off suicide precautions.

If a parent has had her children taken by the child authorities of your state, she is not thinking "I can't be kid-centered when I'm drug-centered." Instead, she is thinking that her world has come to an end. You will want to leave such a person on suicide precautions until she has come to her senses.

It is well known today that drunks kill themselves. Alcoholics and drug addicts are prone to make suicide gestures when someone has walked out on them, no matter how much they deserved it. So you keep them on precautions until they have sobered up.

It is true that jail authorities want to clear people from suicide watch so they have room. But they want more to be free of "successful" suicides. Bottom line: better safe than sorry.

If a person is relaxed and euthymic, she is usually not suicidal. Here is where a complete mental status examination, duly recorded, helps you a lot.

The conditions in which a person on suicide watch is held can be pretty bad. Inmates usually view SW as punitive. You can hardly blame CO's. Rather than call IA, inmates will say they are suicidal to avoid general population. If the conditions are bad enough, inmates will know, and know not just to say they are "suicidal." Thus, unnecessary SW can be prevented through the bad conditions of SW.

If you have any concerns about the safety of an inmate, you can specify conditions in your order. In general, if you have someone on Level 2 (Q15-minute checks), you do not allow him access to clothing, blankets, etc. Even mattresses can be torn and made into ligatures. Our first example was someone on Level 2 that had access to his property. If you are willing to let an inmate have access to normal belongings, then that inmate should be with others. Not only will that provide a witness to suicidal behaviors, but will relieve a borderline's distress at being alone.

There are a variety of approaches to suicidal ideation (SI). For inmates without offspring, you can note that with scientific progress we are on the verge of defeating the aging process. If you are young now, you will probably not get old. You will have time to outlive the consequences of your mistakes. Who cares what you did in your first hundred years if you live to 100,000? Start correcting those mistakes now. In terms of losses, do you think you will still be sad a thousand years in the future for the losses you have suffered today? You will hardly remember your first hundred years. You will certainly not want to end your life when it has hardly started.

If the inmate is a parent, even a non-custodial parent, killing yourself when you still have children means that no one will stand up for them, no one will protect them, no one will advocate for them. Children whose parents committed suicide feel their parents abandoned them. Finally, they feel somehow responsible for the suicide, that they were somehow so unlovable that their parent killed herself.

Suicide

CO's When an inmate completes a suicide, it is a traumatic event both for CO's and involved (living) inmates. CO's should have their own resources available through their EAP. This will probably involve a critical debriefing at the least. It may be your company will provide a psychologist for this, perhaps even the resident psychologist. But don't get involved yourself. Treatment may be provided through the EAP. In any case, there is no medication you can responsibly prescribe for a CO's PTSD.

Inmates may see a dead body before staff can either move it or provide sight barriers. Or an inmate may lose a cellmate or a friend. They may have issues to discuss. Whatever the issues, there are no chemical treatments for PTSD or grief. Any acute medication you would like to prescribe is a drug. You cannot prescribe one of those. Instead, let the staff psychologist or mental health counselors counsel the affected inmates.

Someday enough may be known of treating acute stress to justify prescribing propranolol or other medication. But not yet. And meds carry the potential for side effects.

First of all and last of all, do no harm.

Index

(**Bolded** items are part of section headers)

B

D

G

H

I

N

O

P

S

About the Author

Edward Hume MD JD has practiced psychiatry for more than forty years. Most of the last 17 years he has practiced in jails, with a little time in prisons and a few years in a state hospital.